SEM Micrograph of the
complex trabeculated
inner side of the apex
in a rat right ventricle
from
Endocardial Endothelium:
Functional Morphology
by
Luc J. Andries
© R.G. Landes Co 1994, 1995

MEDICAL
INTELLIGENCE
UNIT

SUDDEN DEATH IN ISCHEMIC HEART DISEASE
AN ALTERNATIVE VIEW ON THE SIGNIFICANCE OF MORPHOLOGIC FINDINGS

Giorgio Baroldi M.D., FACC, FESC
University of Milan
Milan, Italy

Malcolm D. Silver M.D., Ph.D., FRCPA, FRCPC
University of Toronto
Toronto, Ontario, Canada

Springer
New York Berlin Heidelberg London Paris
Tokyo Hong Kong Barcelona Budapest

R.G. LANDES COMPANY
AUSTIN

MEDICAL INTELLIGENCE UNIT

SUDDEN DEATH IN ISCHEMIC HEART DISEASE

R.G. LANDES COMPANY
Austin, Texas, U.S.A.

U.S. and Canada Copyright © 1995 R.G. Landes Company
All rights reserved. Printed in the U.S.A.

Please address all inquiries to the Publisher:
R.G. Landes Company, 909 Pine Street, Georgetown, Texas, U.S.A. 78626
or
P.O. Box 4858, Austin, Texas, U.S.A. 78765
Phone: 512/ 863 7762; FAX: 512/ 863 0081

U.S. and Canada ISBN 1-57059-267-5

International Copyright © 1995 Springer-Verlag, Heidelberg, Germany
All rights reserved.

International ISBN 3-540-59499-X

While the authors, editors and publisher believe that drug selection and dosage and the specifications and usage of equipment and devices, as set forth in this book, are in accord with current recommendations and practice at the time of publication, they make no warranty, expressed or implied, with respect to material described in this book. In view of the ongoing research, equipment development, changes in governmental regulations and the rapid accumulation of information relating to the biomedical sciences, the reader is urged to carefully review and evaluate the information provided herein.

Library of Congress Cataloging-in-Publication Data

Baroldi, Giorgio.
    Sudden death in ischemic heart disease / Giorgio Baroldi, Malcom Silver.
        p. cm. — (Medical intelligence unit)
    Includes bibliographical references and index.
    ISBN 1-57059-267-5 (alk. paper)
    1. Cardiac arrest. 2. Coronary heart disease—Complications.
I. Silver, Malcolm D. II. Title. III. Series.
        [DNLM: 1. Myocardial Ischemia—physiopathology—case studies. 2. Death, Sudden, Cardiac—etiology. WI 300 B264s 1995]
RC685.C173B37 1995
616.1'23025—dc20
DNLM/DLC
for Library of Congress   95-16590
                                                                                          CIP

PUBLISHER'S NOTE

R.G. Landes Company publishes five book series: *Medical Intelligence Unit, Molecular Biology Intelligence Unit, Neuroscience Intelligence Unit, Tissue Engineering Intelligence Unit* and *Biotechnology Intelligence Unit*. The authors of our books are acknowledged leaders in their fields and the topics are unique. Almost without exception, no other similar books exist on these topics.

Our goal is to publish books in important and rapidly changing areas of medicine for sophisticated researchers and clinicians. To achieve this goal, we have accelerated our publishing program to conform to the fast pace in which information grows in biomedical science. Most of our books are published within 90 to 120 days of receipt of the manuscript. We would like to thank our readers for their continuing interest and welcome any comments or suggestions they may have for future books.

Deborah Muir Molsberry
Publications Director
R.G. Landes Company

DEDICATION

To our critics and those we have criticized.

CONTENTS

PREFACE

For millennia *mors subita* (sudden death) was more a voodoo/religious concept than a pathologic problem. Cases are reported in ancient writings. For example and as far as we know, Phidippides was the first "marathon runner" to die suddenly and unexpectedly in 490 B.C. Yet, the frequency of this phenomenon and its link to heart disease were not established. That came with the publication in 1707 of *De Subitaneis Mortibus* prompted by an "epidemic" of sudden death in 1705 at Rome. The latter event so impressed Pope Clement XI that he ordered his "archiatra" or Chief of Medicine, Lancisi, to inquire into the phenomenon. In Lancisi's publication, the first scientific report based on autopsy findings, sudden death was frequently linked to the heart. Subsequently, sudden death as part of ischemic heart disease was recognized as a modern epidemic in frequency and one that particularly affects affluent/consumer societies. Do similarities exist between the 18th century Roman epidemic and the modern one? At best, relationships seem tenuous. Modern societies are populous, rich and technologically advanced while Rome in 1700 was at a peak of decadence and poverty with a small, technologically unsophisticated population. A possible common denominator of the two, apparently opposite, social patterns might be mental depression consequent to loss of hope. Yet, both societies face/faced tension, stresses and depression. Eliot (1994) has reported an epidemic of sudden death amongst NASA (National Aeronautics and Space Administration) employees when, in 1968 the agency faced budget cuts with the loss of highly technical jobs not readily available in other industries. This caused environmental instability.

Modern medical scientists, like their colleague Lancisi, have a duty to discover the genetic, environmental and other factors that cause diseases, or this current epidemic of sudden death. We live in an era of specialists each of whom is elaborately and expensively trained to do only one thing and to act and report on it. People capable of synthesis seem infrequent in science because of this prevalence of specialization. The latter is seen as "a means of institutionalizing, justifying and paying highly for the disintegration of the various functions of character: workmanship, care, conscience and responsibility" (Berry, 1977). A calamity which affects medical science too. One may cite many examples of focally gained knowledge presented as technologic "windows" or "break-throughs" that claim to resolve a problem. They may help to do so, but only when their role is fully assimilated into the overall complexity of a problem.

This book aims to review the pathological findings in sudden "coronary" death comparing them with those found in other forms of acute ischemic disease (myocardial infarction, unstable angina) and with the chronic ischemic syndrome.

It is written more for clinicians than pathologists and integrates our findings with those of many other "images" of ischemic heart disease gained by other specialists. In this it attempts to convert static images into a dynamic process to allow a rational reconstruction of the natural history of ischemic heart disease in all of its acute and chronic syndromes.

The first chapter presents our findings during more than 40 years of morphological investigation, done at first class centers of cardiology practice where application of that expertise allows an easier selection and classification of cases. The second chapter is a compendium of findings on sudden death reported in the literature by others, without any comment or comparison with our data. The third chapter outlines current viewpoints on the natural history of sudden death and ischemic heart disease considering each morphologic variable presumed to have a pathogenic role. The fourth and fifth chapters review the functional significance of arterial and myocardial lesions in relation to current theoretical interpretations. In these sections we compare and contrast our viewpoints with those of others.

Data from our investigations support the following interpretations:

1. Coronary atherosclerotic plaque rupture, thrombosis and embolization are phenomena secondary to myocardial infarct necrosis and to hemodynamic changes following an increased intramyocardial peripheral resistance, i.e., primary myocardial asynergy with stretching of noncontracting myocardium and blockage of intramural flow by intraventricular pressure.

2. The first episode of ischemic heart disease occurs in apparently healthy people, most of whom have one or more severe coronary stenoses of long standing. The lack of previous symptoms and signs confirms the functional adequacy of coronary collaterals demonstrated postmortem. The first episode seems independent of collateral compensation.

3. Atherosclerotic plaque rupture and thrombosis do not happen in small plaques without significant luminal stenosis.

4. No relationship exists between the size of infarct necrosis and complications/death. Also, the concept of "expansion" of an infarct in man is probably a myth.

5. The recognition of other structural forms of myocardial necrosis is vital to determine other pathogenic mechanisms in ischemic heart disease.

6. Two types of coronary atherosclerotic plaque exist, each with a different natural history and progression. One, caused by smooth muscle hyperplasia, is observed in the majority of the population we

studied including those who did not have ischemic heart disease; the other, characterized by subendothelial infiltration of lipid, is related to plaques found in experimental or human familial or acquired hyperlipidemia.

7. Lymphocyte and plasma cell adventitial infiltrates around nerves adjacent to the coronary media act as a possible trigger of pathogenic mechanisms (regional asynergy and/or spasm). Such "active plaques" should be considered in the pathogenesis of ischemic heart disease.

This book is written with two concepts in mind. The first is Donald's (1974), "the value of any investigation may lie more in the questions it raises than in those it answers." The second is that any present pathogenetic theory of ischemic heart disease is just that, a hypothesis. Progress to ultimate knowledge and disease prevention requires an accretion of facts and an intellectual challenge in which both agonists and antagonists are needed.

Acknowledgments

We thank all our co-workers in the different research protocols and in particular, statisticians Fabio Mariani and Gabriella Giuliani and our secretaries Elisabetta Spagnolo and Diana Houghton. Grants were received from the Ontario Heart and Stroke Foundation and Targeted project FATMA, National Research Council, Rome.

Through computer technology Thomas Dearie, Delphi Creative Communications and Dr. Irving Dardick translated 35 mm photographs to the color illustrations in the book. Finally, we are grateful to Fiorella Baroldi and Meredith Silver.

INTRODUCTION

I n the course of evolution, mankind has always paid a high price to survive. Infectious diseases and malnutrition were, and in many areas of the world still are, the main causes of morbidity and death. Where an agricultural lifestyle has been radically changed to the complex technologic/economic system of an affluent society, infectious diseases and malnutrition have been replaced as the major causes of morbidity and death by the "heart attack" usually referred to as coronary or ischemic heart disease. Also, ischemic heart disease generally involves the more competent and competitive people at the time of their highest productivity ("society has need of such men, produces them and destroys them," Morris et al, 1969). Men have long been the chief victims; unfortunately women, too, show increasing propensity to have heart attacks. The resultant socio-economic damage is incalculable as stressed, perhaps too pessimistically, in a 1972 World Health Organization (WHO) report, "... further evolution of the world population in the line of the present technological affluent societies, with increasing economic advances, are in a vicious circle of self-destruction if prevention of ischemic heart disease on a mass scale is not achieved within the next two decades." Those decades have passed yet mortality associated with acute coronary syndromes has been reduced in only a few nations. Ischemic heart disease remains the prime biomedical problem in Western countries. In Italy, for example, of approximately 500,000 deaths per year, 200,000 are of cardiovascular origin, mostly due to ischemic heart disease. Of the latter about half are sudden deaths and occur in people between 40 and 65 years of age (Baroldi, 1985b). In the United States, 500,000 to 600,000 sudden natural deaths are estimated to occur each year, most of which (about 90%) are related to ischemic heart disease (Lie, 1991).

In the past and when dealing with infectious epidemics in the dark ages, the first defense was to identify sources of contagion and isolate them. The main identified risk factors were contact with sick people and infected water, food, etc. The main preventive measure was the lazaret, because of limited therapeutic means. This ghetto prevention reduced, in some way, the *genius morbi*. True preventive and therapeutic measures began only when the etiology of an infectious disease was discovered and immunization or anti-agent medicaments became available.

Despite much knowledge, some of which may prove to be dogma, we are still in the dark ages as far as the cause of ischemic heart disease is concerned. Its pathogenesis is not known exactly, therapy is inadequate to obtain *restitutium ad integrum* and prevention is limited to the identification and reduction of risk factors. Bear in mind that such factors are not necessarily the cause of a disease but only predict risk. We need to know the cause of ischemic heart disease and to prevent it.

The term *acute* ischemic heart disease encompasses different types of angina pectoris and both myocardial infarction and sudden death, the three clinically acute patterns of this disease. Most cases of ischemic heart disease are related to stenosis or occlusion of the lumen of a coronary artery (or of coronary arteries). We note that ischemic heart disease may, in rare instances, be caused by vascular spasm or diseases not related to coronary atherosclerosis. Nevertheless, the concepts that coronary atherosclerotic plaques causing *critical* lumen reduction; acute coronary occlusion by thrombosis following rupture of an atherosclerotic plaque and/or microembolization, with microinfarction are current tenets of pathogenesis. For example, Gorlin and colleagues (1986) commented, "Evidence from serial coronary arteriography and that obtained after reperfusion by thrombolysis, at operation during acute coronary syndromes and from postmortem arteriography have also confirmed the importance of plaque disruption and thrombosis. Indeed, these acute or subacute changes in coronary arterial anatomy appear to be the most frequent cause of all the acute coronary syndromes including unstable angina, myocardial infarction and ischemic sudden death. If we accept the premise that all three acute coronary syndromes may evolve from acute plaque disruption followed by thrombosis or spasm or both, we can construct a unifying theory." The other main clinical pattern of ischemic heart disease is its *chronic* course ending in heart failure as a result of recurrent, nonfatal episodes.

The term *sudden* includes two concepts: one is *chronological*, in the sense of a death which occurs in a short time; the other is *precognitive* because of a lack of symptoms or signs of incipient death; therefore, the death is also *unexpected*. Already, by 1707, in his report Lancisi clearly defined different types of death:

"Huiusmodi vero absoluta cessatio motuum animalium & abscessio animae a corpore, quanquam cogitatione citius perpetua contingant; nihilominus tamen, vulgaris consuetudinis clariorisque doctrinae gratia, mors distinguitur in naturalem, immaturam, & violentam; singulae vero in lentas, & subitaneas, in praevisas, ac praesensas, denique in improvisas, insensiles, atque inopinatas." "Indeed this absolutely complete cessation of animal movements and this departure of the soul from the body, even though it happens at all times more swiftly than thought itself, is nevertheless divided for the sake of common parlance and for greater clarity of teaching, into natural, untimely and violent death, and those again individually into slow and sudden death, into those that are foreseen and forefelt and finally into such as are unforeseen, imperceptible and unexpected" (White et al, 1970).

Lancisi's clear-cut and still up-to-date classification, needs a few comments. First, the meaning of *natural* versus *violent* may be ambiguous. Natural is anything that happens in the natural history of being. This is a very broad concept which may comprise any category of death, including that secondary to violence. Perhaps we should distinguish the following types of death:

1. *Physiological death,* an end result of physiological aging. We do not know its mechanisms and are often unable to discriminate physiological age changes from those of chronic diseases.
2. *Pathological,* or after Lancisi, *natural* death due to diseases including malnutrition/starvation.
3. *Accidental or violent death* due to trauma or any equivalent, e.g., wounding, poisoning, etc., affecting healthy subjects.
4. *Unexplained death* when both clinical and postmortem findings are negative or insufficient to explain its cause.

Lancisi's statement: *"Non utilis modo, sed maxime necessaria Medicis videtur scientia praecognitionis repentinarum mortium, cum nostrae (a) Praeceptor Artis clare ostendat, eum non solum culpa vacaturum, verum etiam boni Medici nomen, atque admirationem consecuturum, qui, cum omnes sanos facere non possit, futura saltem praesentiat atque praedicat."* "The science of the precognition of sudden deaths is seen to be not merely useful but extremely necessary to physicians, since the teacher of our Art (Hippocrates) clearly shows that man not only absolves himself from all blame, but acquires the name of and the admiration owed to a good physician, when he, unable to make everyone well, at least divines and foretells what is about to happen" (White et al, 1970) is an invitation to establish more precisely the frequency of sudden death in any disease.

Among many definitions of sudden death reported in the literature, the following present various points of view:

"... rapid and unforeseen termination of an acute or chronic disease which has in most cases developed in a latent manner" (Brouardel et al, 1902).

"An individual who died due to natural cause and who was not restricted to his house, hospital or other institutions and who was able to function in the community 24 hours prior of death. The time interval for the onset of the fatal event even until death was less than 24 hours" (Kuller et al, 1975).

"Death occurring within one hour, 'early' within 24 hours" (Fulton et al, 1969).

"Instantaneous death within 30 seconds, sudden death in minutes to 24 hours" (Friedman et al, 1973).

"We take the colloquial definition 'sudden' meaning an unexpected or unusual death which was sudden in general terms and which may or may not have been witnessed, but which poses a mystery for explanation" (James, 1973a).

"Witnessed death within one hour of the onset of acute symptoms" (Goldstein, 1982).

" A natural (i.e., nontraumatic) event that is known to have occurred within one hour of the onset of symptoms in a previously healthy person. Use of the term in any other way (to include persons dying , e.g., up to 24 hours after the onset of symptoms) must state the definition explicitly and completely (Hackel et al, 1993).

In outlining a definition of sudden death, the question is whether we really need to establish chronological boundaries. *Survival time*, i.e., the period between the onset of symptoms and death is considered a discriminative parameter in most of the preceding definitions. Timing the fatal episode is obviously important in relation to other variables, to help understand pathogenic mechanisms and their sequence. However, to include or exclude cases based on this parameter seems unjustified, if not misleading. In the present era of emergency hospital services to allow a 24 hour period before death is too long, because adequate clinical investigation could be carried out in that period. On the other hand, death in a 30 second period can be determined only in very limited circumstances; while one hour or even less may be sufficient for a clinical diagnosis on a patient in hospital and two hours may not be enough to do so for a subject who is out-of-hospital. Accordingly the parameter "survival time" was not included in the criteria of selection (see below) in our sudden coronary death study.

Two basic notions pertain to sudden death. First, its mystery from the clinical standpoint. Second, its occurrence in apparently healthy people as well as in those in various phases of a clinically recognized disease; a distinction that any study of sudden death should consider, to gain more precise knowledge of this phenomenon. In term of expectancy, sudden death in a "healthy" marathon runner during a race may be quite different from sudden death in a patient with chronic ischemic heart disease. In other words, a correct approach would distinguish between a *first episode* and a *secondary* event in which complications and/or iatrogenic effects may change the natural history of a disease.

On that basis the definition of sudden death which we prefer is a death that is *rapid (without any specific chronologic limit) and unexpected or unforeseen—both subjectively and objectively—which occurs without any clinical evaluation and in apparently healthy people (primary or unexpected or nonforeseeable sudden death) or in patients during an apparently benign phase in the course of a disease (secondary or expected or foreseeable sudden death)*. Keep in mind that in the present etiologic and pathogenic uncertainty, any definition is only a working one and helps a better selection of material for study. At present uniquely objective data are postmortem findings and, in a select group, electrocardiographic changes in monitored patients or clinical follow-up in people resuscitated from sudden death.

A variety of pathologic conditions may lead to sudden death. Among cardiogenic causes the most frequent is so called *sudden coronary death*. For instance, among 765 out-of-hospital sudden pathological or natural deaths from which our material was selected, 606 were determined by the coroner at autopsy to be due to "coronary disease," namely atherosclerotic obstructive lesions of the coronary arteries; 2 to congenital heart disease and 2 to rheumatic heart disease; 27 had an aortic rupture following intramural dissection; 72 had an acute brain infarct and/or hemorrhage and 56 died of a variety of noncardiovascular conditions (e.g., pneumonia, rupture of esophageal varices in liver cirrhosis, etc.).

The term *sudden coronary death* is in harmony with the classic pathogenic viewpoint, that any coronary arterial obstructive lesion leads to myocardial ischemia with consequent structural and functional damage to the cardiac pump. Already, in 1761, Morgagni had correlated obstructive change of the coronary arteries with chest pain.

═══ CHAPTER 1 ═══

PERSONAL STUDIES

COMPARATIVE PATHOLOGICAL STUDY IN DIFFERENT CLINICAL PATTERNS OF FATAL ISCHEMIC HEART DISEASE

MATERIAL AND CRITERIA FOR SELECTING CASES

The following were studied in our series:

1. Sudden unexpected coronary death (SD)

Two hundred and eight cases of natural primary or nonforeseeable sudden death were studied.

2. Ninety seven cases of accidental death (AD) in normal subjects

These were caused by trauma in 75 instances or carbon monoxide poisoning in 22. All of the foregoing were consecutive cases selected at the Forensic Institute of the Medical School of the University of Milan according to the following criteria:

    a. All SD and the 75 trauma cases were witnessed and occurred outside hospital. The 22 poisoned by carbon monoxide were found dead at home.

    b. A reliable family and personal history was obtained by careful interview of witnesses and family members.

    c. Subjects were participating in normal and usual activity and were not under medical care or taking drugs for any reason. They had no history of any manifest disease which could be related to death and did not received any medical assistance, therapy or resuscitation attempts during the final episode—see following page.

    d. Amongst SD cases significant postmortem findings were absent in all organs other than the heart; the only cardiac lesions being demonstrated at autopsy were coronary atherosclerotic plaques with lumen reduction of some degree and/or myocardial necrosis or fibrosis with or without cardiac hypertrophy.

e. In all SD and trauma cases tests for other poisons or in-
toxicants as a cause of death were negative.

The main reasons why only untreated and apparently healthy subjects were selected for the SD study was firstly, to avoid any superimposed iatrogenic effect due to therapeutic maneuvers and secondly, to
observe phenomena at their earliest without complications due to other
secondary acute or chronic events. The main criticism of this type of
selection is that clinical information (family and personal histories) is
limited and questionable both because of a nonqualified source and
the frequent habit of subjects to minimize or equivocate symptoms.
However, on directly questioning members of the family, in 102 SD
subjects previous minor episodes (chest/arm pain, dyspnea, arm
paresthesia, vertigo), suggestive of latent ischemic heart disease, were
indicated. This group, which apparently had prodomata was arbitrarily
defined as sudden *foreseeable* or *expected* sudden death (SED) and distinguished from the other 106 subjects who died suddenly without
prodromata (sudden *nonforeseeable* or *unexpected* death (SUD), (Baroldi
et al, 1979).

3. Acute myocardial infarction (AMI)

Two hundred consecutive cases of acute myocardial infarction (100
at the Medical School, University of Milan, Italy and 100 at the Toronto
Hospital, Canada) were studied. All had the clinical diagnosis established in a coronary care unit by alterations in ECG tracings and blood
enzyme levels including isoenzymes. No patient had another form of
heart disease or developed the infarction as a complication of a clinical or surgical procedure and none had coronary vascular surgery,
angioplasty or severe resuscitation attempts. All hearts at postmortem
showed histologic evidence of infarct necrosis with an associated polymorphonuclear leukocyte infiltration. Thus, patients were selected for
study only if they had unequivocal clinical and histological evidence
of a myocardial infarction without other diseases and/or iatrogenic
damage.

In order to discriminate between primary and secondary morphologic
alterations a further distinction was made by distinguishing AMI and
SD cases with, and without, extensive ($\geq$ 10 % of the left ventricular
mass) myocardial fibrosis. The latter was considered an acceptable hallmark of previous ischemia. Subjects without extensive myocardial fibrosis were defined *1st episode* of ischemic heart disease and those with
extensive myocardial fibrosis as *2nd episode* of ischemic heart disease.

4. Chronic ischemic heart disease

This group comprised 50 patients, all of whom died at the Toronto
Hospital within 25 days of aortocoronary bypass vein graft surgery for
clinically documented ischemic heart disease with angina pectoris. In
all cases death was caused by congestive heart failure.

5. Noncardiac diseases

These included 140 patients dead of noncardiac diseases (brain infarction/hemorrhage, pneumonia, etc.) at Milan University Hospital. (Baroldi et al, 1974; Silver et al, 1980).

METHOD OF EXAMINING THE HEART

In all cases an autopsy was performed between 14 and 74 hours of death, the body being refrigerated at 4°C before examination.

All organs, the aorta and its main branches were carefully examined. The heart was removed from the body, washed and weighed. It was then fixed undistended for 24 hours in 10% buffered formaldehyde solution. After mild fixation coronary arteries and their main branches distributed on the surface of the heart (*extramural* or *epicardial coronary arteries* or *branches*) were cross sectioned at 3 mm intervals along their whole course. Samples for histologic examination were taken systematically at the origin of left main coronary artery (LMA), left anterior descending branch (LADB), left circumflex branch (LCXB), right coronary artery (RCA), posterior descending branch (PDB), second distal LADB and at the marginal and middle portion of the posterior tract of the RCA. Furthermore, all 3 mm cross sections of any stenoses seen by the naked eye were sampled for histology. All samples were placed in 10% buffered formalin to complete fixation and decalcified when needed.

Each heart was cut by a machine into slices 1 cm thick parallel to the posterior atrioventricular groove and proceeding from apex to base, with the last section at the upper level of the left ventricular papillary muscles, usually 3-4 cm from the atrioventricular groove. After another 24 hours fixation, sliced hearts were examined and the location, type and size of any myocardial damage recorded. Photographs of the slices, made on a grid divided into 1 cm squares, were enlarged and any areas of acute infarction or fibrosis and the total area of each slice were measured using a polar planimeter. In this manner, the size of an infarct or scar, expressed as a percentage of total left ventricular mass including the whole septum was calculated. Histologic sections were used to establish the edges of an infarct or scar when assessing the affected area.

In each heart the entire (2 cm x whole wall thickness) ventricular wall at the basal, median and apical levels of the anterior, lateral and posterior walls of both left and right ventricles, the anterior and posterior left and right papillary muscles, the anterior and posterior interventricular septum and the left and right atria were examined histologically. Furthermore, any naked eye lesion in the myocardium was estimated and sampled for histology. An average of 40 sections from 18 different areas were examined per heart. Both coronary arteries and myocardium were stained with hematoxylin and eosin; when necessary Movat pentachrome, Weigert elastic, Mallory and PAS stains were employed.

In sudden death cases the conduction system was excised according to the methods of Lev et al, (1951, 1954). Systematic samples were taken of the sinus node, the atrio-ventricular node, His bundle and its branches.

The 100 AMI hearts studied at the Toronto Hospital had a post-mortem injection of barium sulphate (Micropaque, Damancy and Co., Slough, UK) in the coronary arteries at a pressure of 120 mm Hg. Radiographic images were made in the anteroposterior and both left and right anterior oblique views.

ANALYSIS OF EXTRAMURAL CORONARY ARTERIES

Physical variables

In all histologic sections of coronary arteries the following parameters were evaluated:

Intimal and medial thickness

The maximal intimal thickness was measured histologically in microns by a micrometer. Minimal and maximal thicknesses of the media were established in the same manner and a ratio "maximal/minimal medial width x 50" was calculated. We distinguished the following types of intimal thickening: (1) a *physiologic* one; (2) that observed in *atherosclerosis* and (3) a non*atherosclerotic obstructive* intimal thickening (see chapter 3 for definitions).

Lumen reduction by atherosclerotic plaque

The degree of lumen reduction found histologically in a coronary artery was expressed as a percentage and measured as a reduction in luminal diameter. This method was chosen in preference to measuring the cross sectional area because an atherosclerotic plaque may distend a vessel wall. The rationale is to compare the normal lumen of a vessel with the residual one. The major and minor diameters of the residual lumen were measured in each section of a coronary artery using a micrometer and the results averaged. That average diameter was related to the average luminal diameter obtained in a plastic cast study of coronary arteries from normal hearts (see below; Baroldi et al, 1967).

We are aware that no method of establishing the degree of a coronary artery stenosis is entirely satisfactory. When postmortem injection is not performed a criticism is the lack of fixation of vessels under pressure. We noted no significant difference in the distribution of the degree and number of stenoses found in two series of 100 AMI cases one *without,* (Baroldi et al, 1974) and the other *with,* postmortem coronary injection under pressure followed by fixation (Silver et al, 1980); (Table 1). What is needed is a reproducible method that permits comparison between different populations to establish the trend of variable "lumen reduction."

Table 1. *Maximal lumen diameter reduction and number of vessels with severe (≥ 70%) stenosis in acute infarct cases without and with postmortem fixation of coronary arteries under pressure**

AMI cases	Maximal lumen reduction %				No. of vessels ≥70% stenosis		
	≤69	70	80	≥90	1	2	3
100 without	11	20	27	42	38	36	15
100 with pressure	6	18	29	47	39	35	20
Total	17	38	56	89	77	71	35

a $c^2_3 = 1.93$ P> 0.05
b $c^2_2 = 0.61$ P> 0.05

* see text for details

Luminal stenosis

A luminal stenosis in a coronary artery was defined as being *severe, functional* or *critical,* i.e., capable of reducing flow when it was equal to, or more than, 70% (a 70% lumen/diameter stenosis roughly corresponds to a 90% lumen/area stenosis). The stenosis was *mild* when lumen reduction was less than 70% lumen/diameter. To compare stenoses in each main vessel among groups with different causes of death the *maximal lumen reduction* found in a vessel was considered. This allowed us to evaluate any degree of stenosis in one or more main vessels against several parameters (e.g., infarct size, survival, etc.). In most tables different degrees of a luminal stenosis are reported.

Length of stenosis

The length of a maximal luminal stenosis in the gross was calculated in millimeters by judging its extension into sequential 3 mm cross sections of the vessel.

Type of stenosis

Histologically a luminal stenosis was defined as *concentric,* either when the residual lumen was centrally located or when it was lateral but still encircled by pathologic tissue or *semilunar,* when part of the arterial wall was normal.

Luminal occlusion

Thrombus

In its early stage a thrombus (*acute thrombus*) is mainly composed of platelet aggregates, fibrin and some polymorphonuclear leukocytes; later, in healing, it shows different stages of organization with eventual luminal fibrosis and recanalization (*old thrombus*).

Occlusive thrombus

We included in this category any thrombus that "completely" occluded a coronary artery lumen. The morphology of a thrombus may change with location in the lumen, being completely occlusive in one section and partially occlusive (75%) in another (e.g., in its "tail"). Because of this we included partially occlusive with completely occlusive thrombi.

Mural thrombus

Such thrombi occluded less than 50% of the lumen. In general, *acute mural thrombi* were formed by thin, mainly fibrinous, lamina which did not reduce the lumen significantly. *Old mural thrombi* showed different stages of organization.

Morphologic variables

TYPE OF ATHEROSCLEROTIC PLAQUE: A plaque was defined as *atheromatous* or *fibrous* according to whether atheromatous material or fibrous tissue (without basophilia and/or atheroma) predominated in it. The following variables were also defined and considered:

BASOPHILIA is a pale, amorphous basophilic substance produced by proteoglycan accumulation without cellular reaction. It is generally found in the deeper layer of the thickened intima of a fibrous plaque.

ATHEROMA consisted of a combination of lipoprotein material, foam cells and crystalline, cholesterol clefts.

CALCIFICATION formed by basophilic granules of various size or as a plaque of darkly basophilic material replacing intimal tissue.

INTIMAL HEMORRHAGE was indicated by extravascular red blood cells found in lesions in various amounts.

All of the above variables were defined as being *mild* when, in total, an individual one involved one-quarter or less of the circumference of the vessel wall; *moderate* if half was involved and *severe* if more than half of the circumference was affected.

INTIMAL VASCULARIZATION was characterized by finding capillary-like, newly formed, vessels of various diameter in the thickened intima. According to their number, vascularization was considered *mild* if less than three lumina were seen, *moderate* if four to six or *extensive* if more than six.

INTIMAL AND ADVENTITIAL LYMPHOCYTIC INFILTRATION was marked by inflammatory cells, mainly small lymphocytes and plasma cells in the intima or adventitia. Only occasionally was an infiltrate granulomatous and showed giant cells. An inflammatory reaction whether or not with granulomatous features was considered *mild* when only a few, scattered cellular elements were found, *moderate* when few but well profiled foci of lymphocytes were present and *severe* when a massive inflammatory reaction was seen (Baroldi et al, 1988).

ANALYSIS OF INTRAMURAL CORONARY ARTERIES

In each histologic myocardial section the status of *intramural* or *intramyocardial* vascular branches of any type, including the terminal bed and veins was investigated. The following main structural changes were considered:

Emboli

PLATELET AGGREGATES in a vessel lumen consist of unstained granular material, formed by very small, roundish elements with different degrees of aggregation or often affected by partial lytic dissolution. No demonstrable fibrin was associated with them.

To calculate their frequency 16 histologic sections of myocardium (5 left ventricle, 5 right ventricle, 4 interventricular septum and 1 for each atrium) were selected at random from all histologic slides of each sudden and accidental death case. They included the sinus node in 120 SD and 63 AD cases and the AV-node bundle of His in 180 and 95 cases respectively. In each section the number of arterial intramural vessels partially ($\geq$70% of the lumen) or completely occluded by platelet aggregates were counted by screening the entire section at 250 x magnification. A total of 3328 sections in 208 SD, and 1552 in 97 AD groups were examined (Baroldi et al, 1980). The presence or absence of venous platelet aggregates and blood stasis was also estimated.

FIBRIN/PLATELET THROMBI OR EMBOLI are constituted by an association, in variable proportion, of fibrin and platelets. They may form in situ *(thrombi)* or have origin from a proximal source *(emboli)*.

Vascular stasis

Due to postmortem changes and technical artifacts it is difficult to objectively quantify the amount of blood in myocardial tissue. To have a rough estimate of stasis at death, *intramural stasis,* was defined as *arterial* or *venous* or both when in each histological section at least 5 intramural arterial or/and venous vessels respectively were well filled by red blood cells (Baroldi et al, 1980).

Medial hyperplasia obliterans

By this definition we indicate a medial change affecting small intramyocardial vessels. A hyperplastic process with formation of longitudinal bundles of smooth muscle cells found mainly in the outer media that causes luminal stenosis. We consider finding fibrous tissue penetrating into and replacing medial muscular tissue a late stage of this process. Usually intima and internal elastic membrane are normal. Only occasionally fibrous intimal thickening and degenerative alteration of the elastic membrane are seen. The latter, resulting from the medial changes, are more frequent in affected vessels with severe lumen reduction. This pattern was defined as *minimal* when only 1 vessel showing these changes was present in at least 1 of the 18 areas examined, *moderate* when 2 vessels were affected and *severe* when more than 2 vessels were seen (Baroldi, 1986).

ANALYSIS OF MYOCARDIAL CHANGES

Acute myocardial necrosis

The different forms of myocardial necrosis observed in ischemic heart disease and stages in their healing (see Table 2 and chapter 3 "Natural history of myocardial cell necrosis" for details of definitions) were evaluated as follows:

Infarct necrosis was estimated as a percent of the left ventricular mass (see above). *Coagulative myocytolysis* (or *Zenker necrosis*) and *colliquative myocytolysis* (or *myocytolysis*) were judged *minimal* when less than 5 foci were observed in 1 myocardial section, *moderate* when a similar number of foci were seen in 2 or 3 sections and *extensive* when that number was present in 4 or more sections.

Myocardial fibrosis

Myocardial fibrosis was classified as *recent* by the presence of fibroblasts and vessels or *old* when it was dense, hypocellular and avascular scar tissue. It was estimated *minimal* when only a few foci were detected histologically, *moderate* when its extension was less than 10% of the left ventricular mass and *extensive* when more than 10%.

Cardiac hypertrophy

In our material, heart weight was reported in 100 g classes (<200, 200-299, 300-399 g, etc.). However, for comparative purpose and to avoid indices related to body weight and/or height, we adopted Linzbach's distinction (1947) between *physiologic* (<500 g) and *pathologic* (≥500 g) *hypertrophy*. In general, a heart exceeding 500 g has a pathologically increased mass. A heart was defined *atrophic* when it weighed less than 250 g for a man and 200 g for a woman (normal average weight 300 and 250 g respectively, Silver MM et al, 1991).

STATISTICAL ANALYSES

All variables and their ratings were recorded on original cards. The data were processed by an IBM 370/168 computer. Analyses were accomplished by nonparametric tests (Bishop et al, 1980). The significance of first and superior-order associations was investigated by loglinear models. When a "fit" of specific models was obtained, further analysis on the pertinent contingency tables was done by residual and lambda parameter analyses. For subject analysis, chi-square tests and "filling" to binomial distribution function were used. Possible associations among morphological variables were tested, using two codes for comparison. They were: comparing no change versus mild + moderate

Table 2. Histologic pattern in different types of myocardial necrosis in CHD*

Myocardium	Coagulation Necrosis (Infarct Necrosis)	Coagulative Myocytolysis (Zenker Necrosis)	Colliquative Myocytolysis (Myocytolysis)
Functional status	Irreversible relaxation ("atonic" death) + stretching by intraventricular pressure	Irreversible contraction ("tetanic" death)	Progressive loss of function ("failing" death)
Muscle fiber	Early thinning	Normal or swollen	Increasing edema - vacuolization
Nucleus	Elongation-pyknosis progressive karyolysis	Normal	Normal
Myofibrils	Elongated sarcomeres in normal registered order, even in late stage	Rhexis - Anomalous irregular cross band formations (coagulation of hypercontracted sarcomeres)	Progressive disappearance "empty cell" (colliquation)
Vessels	Secondary wall degeneration and thrombosis	Normal	Normal
Infiltration	Massive polymorphonuclear exudation	No early cellular infiltrates. Possible late lymphocytes	No infiltrates
Extension-Location	In general unique massive focus of different size. Subendocardial to transmural	Multiple (mono or pluricellular) disseminated or confluent foci of different size in any area	Focal progressively spreading
Irreversible in	At least 20-60 min	Few minutes	?
Healing	Removal by macrophages. Collagenization of empty sarcolemmal tubes		?
Frequency in IHD: Acute infarct	100%	100% at outer edges of early infarct 85% in myocardium elsewhere	38% subendocardial and perivascular
Sudden death	17% histologically demonstrated	72% (unique demonstrable lesion), 86% (including cases with infarct)	8%

*CHD = Coronary Heart Disease

+ severe changes (sensitive code), and comparing no change + mild change + moderate change vs severe change (specific code). To avoid tedious repetition of chi-square values in the text, a *significant* result indicates one where the P value is <0.05. Also, in the text and tables, numerical results have been rounded with those 0.5 or less reported as the prime number and those greater than 0.5 increased to the next number.

The distinction between sudden death cases with (SED) and without prodromata (SUD) is maintained only in cases of significant statistical differences. Otherwise, all sudden death cases are considered as one group (SD).

OTHER PERTINENT PERSONAL STUDIES

PLASTIC CAST STUDY OF CORONARY VESSELS AND COLLATERALS

Pertinent to the present review is a previous study in which the anatomy of the coronary vascular system was investigated, with particular reference to *collaterals* or *anastomoses* defined as channels joining branches of different arteries. This study included 69 normal adults, 50 who died by accident and 19 from noncardiovascular diseases and 10 children from newborn to 10 years of age who died from noncardiovascular diseases; other adult hearts studied included 25 patients with atrophy and 48 with hypertrophy of the heart, of left or right ventricle or both ventricles, both groups having normal coronary arteries; 18 patients with chronic anemia and/or hypoxic diseases but a normal heart; 217 patients with obstructive lesions of any degree of the coronary arteries; 70 cases of out-of-hospital sudden and unexpected coronary death and 147 hospitalized patients; of the latter, 47 died of acute myocardial infarction, 21 were associated with extensive fibrosis and 100 had a normal myocardium or minimal myocardial fibrosis and died of noncardiac causes. All cases were selected by the same criteria mentioned above in our "comparative pathologic study."

Plastic material (Geon latex 756 or Neoprene 842 A) was injected into coronary arteries through the aorta after hermetically closing the aortic valve. The injected material was solidified by subsequently placing a heart in 10% formalin at 40-50°C for 48-72 hours. Before corroding the organ by concentrated hydrochloric acid solution, myocardial samples from different cardiac areas were secured for histology. The injection of plastic material and subsequent corrosion allowed accurate tridimensional casts of the coronary tree to vessels of 20 μm diameter (Fig. 1). The lack of shrinkage during solidification permitted a correct evaluation of luminal diameter and its reduction when stenosed. The diameter of vessels measured on these casts was considered the diameter in maximal dilation since they were injected and fixed under 120 mm Hg pressure.

The arterial collateral circulation was estimated by an *anastomotic index* (AI) formulated as follows: AI = Max ø +(AV ø x Frequency)/100 in which *Max ø* was the diameter in microns of the largest anastomotic vessel found; *AV ø* was the average diameter of larger anastomoses, greater than 100 μm and *frequency* was the frequency of anastomoses greater than 100 μm found in any heart. In this respect an average of 40 such anastomoses were usual in a normal heart providing an arbitrary index of 1. Collaterals were distinguished as being *homocoronary,* when they connected branches of the same coronary artery or *intercoronary*, when branches of different coronary arteries were joined. *Extracardiac* collaterals ran between coronary branches and other adjacent arterial systems, e.g., bronchial arteries.

Finally, using different techniques of injection, the coronary venous system, including coronary sinus system and anterior cardiac venous system, were studied in 74 cases. Also, the arterioluminal and venoluminal vessels, i.e., connections between coronary arteries and veins and cardiac chambers were investigated in 48 cases and extracardiac arterial connections in 13 cases (Baroldi et al, 1967).

Reviewing these casts, the following patterns of coronary artery distribution were defined: In *type I* (77%) the right coronary artery (RCA) gave rise to the posterior descending branch. According to the length of the RCA three subtypes were recognized. In *type I α (5%)* the RCA ended as soon as it became the posterior descending branch without significant ramification on the posterior left ventricle; in *type I β (55%)* the RCA vascularized half of the posterior left ventricle; in *type I γ (17%)* all of the posterior left ventricle was nourished by the RCA which ended at the left cardiac margin. In *type II* (8%) the posterior descending branch originated from the left circumflex artery and in *type III (15%)* two posterior descending branches existed, one arising from the left circumflex and right coronary arteries respectively. A *third coronary artery,* conus artery or arteria coronaria accessoria dextra was observed in 46% of cases; occasionally, it was doubled (8% of cases) or tripled (1% of cases).

CHRONOLOGICAL RELATIONSHIP
BETWEEN OCCLUSIVE THROMBUS AND INFARCT NECROSIS

Different chronological stages of a coronary thrombus (Irniger, 1963) and myocardial infarct necrosis (Mallory et al, 1939) have been outlined. Accordingly, *coeval* associations between thrombus and infarct necrosis were evaluated histologically in 208 acute infarct cases, 116 "unexpected" and 112 "expected" sudden coronary death all from the files of the Armed Forces Institute of Pathology, Washington DC, USA. The following were related:

1. Early thrombus without vessel wall reaction vs apparently normal myocardium or infarct necrosis with different degrees of polymorphonuclear leukocyte infiltration in the heart muscle.

2. Thrombus with endothelial proliferation/capillary growth
    vs initial macrophagic reaction at the periphery of an infarct.
3. Thrombus with early organization, e.g., collagen fibril depo-
    sition vs diffuse granulomatous-like appearance of myocar-
    dial infarct necrosis.
4. Recent organized thrombus vs recent myocardial fibrosis,
    e.g., numerous fibroblasts and monocytes (Baroldi, 1965).

SMALL VESSEL DISEASE AND MICROCIRUCLATORY IMPAIRMENT IN THE HUMAN HEART

To establish a relationship between platelet or red blood cell ag-
gregations or obstructive small vessel disease and ischemic heart disease, 53 cases of *sickle cell anemia* and 39 of *thrombotic thrombocytopenic
purpura (TTP)* from the files of the Armed Forces Institute of Pathology, Washington, DC., USA were examined. (Baroldi et al, 1967; Baroldi,
1969). In each case clinical and autopsy records and 2 or more samples
of myocardium were available for study. A serial section study of 2
blocks from both cardiac ventricles was done in 3 TTP cases. An average of 200 sections of 8μm thickness were stained by hematoxylin
and eosin.

FINDINGS IN OUR COMPARATIVE PATHOLOGICAL STUDY

PATIENT DATA

Gender and age

Table 3 shows a prevalence of men in the sudden death (SD) group
and amongst controls. This difference was less evident among acute
myocardial infarct (AMI) patients. The highest incidence of sudden
death occurred in the sixth decade for men (P <0.01) and in the eighth
decade for women (P <0.01). AMI had a higher frequency amongst
men in their seventh decade (P <0.05) and amongst women in their
eighth decade (P <0.05).

Both body weight and somatotype were within normal range in
AMI, SD and control subjects.

Survival time

Survival time ranged from 6 hours to 30 days in AMI patients. In
151 SD subjects it was less than 10 minutes, up to 1 hour in 47 and
up to 3 hours in 10. In accidental death (AD) cases death occurred
within 10 minutes in 75 people dying from trauma and in less than 6
hours amongst 22 dying from carbon monoxide poisoning.

Table 3. Sex and age frequency distribution of cases studied personally

		<40	40-49	50-59	60-69	≥70	Total
				Age (years)			
SD	Men	30	31	63*	41	17	182
	Women	5	2	5	4	10*	26
	Total	35	33	68	45	27	208
AMI	Men	4	18	35	45+	36	138
	Women	–	4	9	22	27+	62
	Total	4	22	44	67	63	200
AD	Men	9	11	27	20	21	88
	Women	1	2	1	3	2	9
	Total	10	13	28	23	23	97

Man/Woman ratio: SD = 7; AMI = 2; AD = 10
* $p < 0.01$
+ $p < 0.05$

Activity, cigarette and alcohol use

About half the SD subjects were engaged in an activity when they died suddenly, 52 were at work, 44 walking and 13 driving. The other half were sleeping or resting. The distribution as far as the type of work performed was 60% manual (light 10%, moderate 22%, heavy 28%) and sedentary or executive work in 20% respectively.

Amongst the 208 SD subjects, 28% were nonsmokers, 22% mild cigarette smokers (half package per day) and 49% heavy cigarette smokers (more than one package per day). A similar distribution was seen in AD controls. Alcohol intake was heavy (more than 5 liters of wine per day) in 13% of SD people and 10% in controls. Neither activity at the time of infarct onset nor cigarette and alcohol use were considered in AMI cases.

Extramural Coronary Arteries

All cases included in this study showed a physiological intimal thickening that did not significantly reduce the lumen of extramural or subepicardial coronary arteries. Pathologic intimal thickening seen in our material was atherosclerotic in nature (for definition of different types of intimal thickening see chapter 3).

Atherosclerotic intimal thickening

Degree of lumen reduction, its location and its relationship to age in different groups

Table 4 presents the degrees of luminal stenosis caused by atherosclerosis and the age distribution amongst our 97 normal subjects. Thirty-eight of them proved to have a severe (≥70%) coronary artery stenosis,

Table 4. *Frequency distribution of coronary atherosclerotic stenosing plaques in 97 adult "normal" subjects (88 men - 9 women) dying by accident, without history and post-mortem finding of any disease*

Decades	No. cases	Maximal lumen reduction %*						Stenosis vs No. vessels					
								Any type			Severe (≥70%)		
		0	<50	50-69	70-79	80-89	>90	1	2	3	1	2	3 or more
<39	10	2	3	4	1	–	–	3	3	2	–	1	–
40-49	13	2	6	2	2	1	–	1	5	5	2	1	–
50-59	28	4	7	7	5	4	1	3	6	15	6	3	1
60-69	23	–	2	9	5	4	3	5	3	15	7	4	1
>70	23	–	2	9	6	4	2	–	4	19	7	4	1
Total	97	8	20	31	19	13	6	12	21	56	22	13	3

* % lumen diameter

with such stenoses being present in more than one main vessel in 16. If the 74 subjects in this group who were more than 50 years old are considered, 46% had a severe luminal stenosis. These were at multiple sites in 19%. None of these individuals had clinical ischemic heart disease or moderate/extensive myocardial fibrosis. One notes that 21% and 32% of these subjects had at least one <50% stenosis or a 50-69% stenosis respectively.

Table 5 indicates the behavior of variable "lumen reduction" amongst patients with acute infarction or sudden death or in controls, in relation to their age. The frequency of severe stenosis from 40 to 69 years to ≥70 years of age increased from 90% to 95% in AMI, 39% to 52% in controls and was constant (81%) in SD cases. The increases were not statistically significant. To establish the behavior of atherosclerotic stenoses in relation to previous episodes of ischemic heart disease and other noncardiac diseases, AMI and SD groups were subdivided into patients with their first episode and no extensive myocardial fibrosis and patients with a positive clinical history and myocardial fibrosis greater than 10% of left ventricular mass. Furthermore, the findings in 100 noncardiac patients dying from various diseases of other organs e.g., brain hemorrhage, pneumonia, liver cirrhosis, etc. were compared with AMI, SD and AD groups (Table 6). Data show that a significantly greater frequency of coronary atherosclerotic obstructions are demonstrable in patients with previous ischemic episodes in both AMI and SD groups. Furthermore, death may be independent of the degree of lumen reduction and number of main arteries or branches with severe stenosis; and is less frequent (P < 0.01) in patients with previous ischemic episodes. Of 200 consecutive infarct cases and 208 sudden death cases 72% and 64% respectively died at the first episode of illness.

Table 5. Frequency distribution of maximal lumen reduction and number of vessels with severe stenosis (≥ 70% lumen diameter) in relation to age in sudden coronary death (SD), acute myocardial infarct (AMI) and in healthy subjects dying by accident (AD)

Age yrs	Lumen reduction (%)					Stenosis ≥70% in			
	<69	70-79	80-89	> 90	Total	1	2	3 +	Total
								vessels	
≤ 39									
SD	18*	1	9	7	35	7	6	4	17
AMI	1	2	–	1	4	2	–	1	3
AD	9	1	–	–	10	–	1	–	1
40-69									
SD	28	20	39	59*	146	37	45	36	118
AMI	13	21	37	62*	133	46	50	24	120
AD	39*	12	9	4	64	14	9	2	25
≥ 70									
SD	5	8	5	9*	27	9	9	4	22
AMI	3	15	19	26*	63	29	21	10	60
AD	11	6	4	2	23	8	3	1	12
Total									
SD	51	29	53	75*	208	53	60	44	157
AMI	17	38	56	89*	200	77*	71	35	183
AD	59*	19	13	6	97	22	13	3	38

* P < 0.01

Table 6. Maximal lumen reduction and number of main subepicardial coronary arteries with severe (> 70% lumen diameter) stenosis

Source	No. cases	% Maximal lumen reduction						Severe stenosis in		
		0	< 50	50-69	70-79	80-89	> 90	1	2	3
									vessels	
AMI lst	145	3 (2)	3 (2)	10 (7)	30 (21)	45 (31)	54 (37)	61 (42)	49 (34)	19 (13)
AMI 2nd	55	–	1 (2)	–	8 (14)	11 (20)	35 (64)	16 (29)	22 (40)	16 (29)
Total	200	3 (1)	4 (2)	10 (5)	38 (19)	56 (28)	89 (44)	77 (38)	71 (35)	35 (17)
SD lst	133	10 (8)	18 (13)	18 (13)	21 (16)	39 (29)	27 (20)	40 (30)	34 (25)	13 (10)
SD 2nd	75	–	–	5 (7)	8 (11)	14 (18)	48 (64)	13 (17)	26 (35)	31 (41)
Total	208	10 (5)	18 (9)	23 (11)	29 (14)	53 (25)	75 (36)	53 (25)	60 (29)	44 (21)
NCA	100	7 (5)	10 (10)	17 (17)	11 (11)	24 (24)	31 (31)	26 (26)	18 (18)	22 (22)
AD	97	8 (8)	20 (21)	31 (32)	19 (19)	13 (14)	6 (6)	22 (23)	13 (13)	3 (3)

AMI, acute myocardial infarct; SD, sudden coronary death; NCA, noncardiac atherosclerotic patients; AD, normal subjects dying from accident; lst = first episode and 2nd = two or more episodes of ischemic heart disease.

Amongst all 455 patients with ischemic heart disease the left anterior descending branch in its proximal part was the vessel with the highest frequency of stenoses of any degree (90%) and critical stenoses with lumen/diameter reduction higher than 70% (41%) followed by the anterior segment of the right coronary artery (85% and 35% respectively), proximal portion of the left circumflex branch (74% and 30%), distal portion of left anterior descending branch (68% and 29%), and the marginal (59% and 21%) and posterior (34% and 12%) segments of the right coronary artery. The vessels least frequently involved by any degree of stenosis were the left main trunk (50% all stenoses and 4% severe stenosis) and the posterior descending branch (10% and 3% respectively).

Length of stenosis

In all groups the length of mild stenoses (≤69%) was significantly shorter (≤3 mm) in AMI and SD cases while in chronic IHD the longest (>30 mm) stenoses prevailed; amongst AD subjects, short and long stenoses had the same frequency. In contrast, severe stenoses (≥70%) generally had a significant tendency to increase in length with an increasing degree of lumen reduction. In AMI patients, however, the majority of severe stenoses showed the shortest length (≤3 mm), in contrast to normal controls who mainly presented stenoses with the longest length (≥30 mm). It must be noted that along the course of a stenosis variations of lumen reduction existed.

Type of stenosis

The atherosclerotic plaque at the site of maximal lumen reduction was concentric in 70% and semilunar in 30% of all cases. Semilunar plaques showed a higher association with mild (40%) than severe stenoses (13%).

Morphological variables of the atherosclerotic plaque

Of the 3,640 coronary sections studied, 1,519 had no obvious lumen reduction and an intimal thickness less than 300 μm (*physiological thickening*). In the other 2,121 sections lumen reduction was caused by atherosclerotic plaque.

In the first group without lumen reduction, morphologic atherosclerotic variables were insignificant. Only in 1% were plaques too small to produce any measurable lumen reduction and had minimal histologic changes. A different distribution of plaque variables in relation to the degree of lumen reduction/intimal thickness per se and in different ischemic heart disease groups was observed in the second group (Table 7a and b).

A practical note is that severe intimal calcification was frequently associated (33%) with mild coronary artery stenosis. This means that the angiographic demonstration of coronary calcification, while a hallmark of atherosclerosis, is not necessarily one of severe lumen reduction.

When morphologic variables in plaques with the same lumen reduction and intimal thickness were compared among the different patient groups significant divergencies were noted as follows:

1. Among AMI cases, atheroma, hemorrhage, calcification and lymphocytic and plasma cell infiltrates prevailed, independent of the degree of lumen reduction. In contrast, these variables were significantly less frequent in controls, while chronic ischemia and SD groups had an intermediate position. Chronic ischemic patients were more like acute infarct and sudden death cases than controls.

2. Intimal hemorrhage was the least frequent variable found (14% of total mild and severe plaques). It was mainly observed in severe concentric stenoses located in a vessel related to an acute myocardial infarct.

3. Intimal or adventitial inflammation or both were present in all AMI cases, in the majority of chronic and sudden death cases and significantly less in controls (Table 8). The association of this inflammatory process first with basophilia (Table 9) was equal in all groups. Also, in all groups

Table 7a. Percentage distribution of morphological variables of atherosclerotic and fibrous plaques in relation to lumen reduction and intimal thickness

						Morphological variables					
	Total	Absent	BS	AT	IV	HR	CA	ILI	ALI	ALI+ILI	FP
Lumen reduction (%)											
0	1519	97	0.5	0.3	0.4	0.2	0.2	0.3	0.5	0.9	–
<50	687	34	52	27	31	3	27	26	20	32	45
50-69	632	8	70	54	63	8	48	52	43	62	20
70-79	298	3	71	75	74	19	58	67	54	74	12
80-89	262	1	71	77	82	30	63	69	64	84	9
≥90	242	2	58	74	78	33	69	69	66	82	16
Intimal thickness μm^c											
≤299	162	93	3	2	3	–	3	2	1	2	96
300-599	199	34	50	16	24	1	21	23	14	28	49
600-999	544	8	69	42	57	6	38	45	36	54	24
1000-1.999	926	3	75	69	75	18	60	62	53	73	12
≥2000	290	4	57	76	63	30	64	68	62	79	13

Abbreviations: Absent, no morphologic variables; ALI, adventitial lymphocytic infiltration; AT, atheroma; BS, basophilia; CA, calcification; FP, fibrous plaque without atheroma and/or basophilia; HR, intimal hemorrhage; ILI, intimal lymphocytic infiltration; IV, intimal vascularization.
^{c} Only sections with lumen reduction considered here.

Table 7b. Percentage distribution of morphological variables and of atherosclerotic fibrous plaques in different groups in relation to lumen reduction and intimal thickness[a]

Morphological variables Group (sections)	Absent	FP[a]	BS	AT	IV	HR	CA	ILI	ALI	ILI+ALI
No lumen reduction										
AMI (309)	96	–	2	1	2	1	1	1	2	3
CI (225)	99	–	0.4	–	–	–	0.4	1	–	1
SDP (245)	100	–	0.4	–	0.4	–	–	0.4	–	0.4
SDNP (335)	100	–	0.3	–	–	–	0.3	–	1	1
AD (405)	100	–	–	–	–	–	–	–	–	–
Total (1519)	99	–	0.5	0.3	0.4	0.2	0.3	0.5	0.5	1
Lumen reduction ≤69%										
AMI (264)	9	17	72	56	43	16	50	55	46	67
CI (77)	23	43	40	43	40	9	43	51	40	57
SDP (346)	25	40	54	34	48	2	35	37	26	43
SDNP (325)	22	32	65	41	53	4	36	34	31	42
AD (307)	28	37	59	30	41	2	27	28	20	35
Lumen reduction ≥70%										
AMI (227)	0.4	11	60	78	72	43	74	74	65	85
CI (98)	4	14	44	73	68	32	63	76	67	87
SDP (225)	3	12	76	72	82	21	58	64	65	77
SDNP (188)	2	13	72	76	86	20	61	64	54	75
AD (64)	3	8	80	75	72	8	44	64	42	72
Grand total (2121)	14	25	63	53	58	14	47	50	42	59
Intimal thickness(μm) ≤599										
AMI (43)	26	39	58	21	28	5	21	39	21	44
CI (3)	33	67	33	33	67	–	–	67	33	67
SDP (105)	69	80	19	9	10	–	9	11	4	13
SDNP (98)	59	72	26	9	13	–	16	10	9.	13
AD (112)	66	71	28	6	12	–	11	6	6	9
Intimal thickness (μm) ≥600										
AMI (448)	3	12	67	71	59	31	65	66	58	78
CI (172)	12	26	42	60	56	22	55	65	56	74
SDP (466)	4	18	72	58	73	11	52	56	50	66
SDNP (415)	4	14	78	65	78	12	52	53	47	64
AD (259)	5	15	77	52	61	4	39	46	32	55

[a]Only sections with lumen reduction considered here.
[b]Abbreviations: AD, accidental death; ALI, adventitial lymphocytic infiltration; AMI, acute myocardial infarction; AT, atheroma; BS, basophilia; CA, calcification; CI, chronic ischemia; FP, fibrous plaque without atheroma and/or basophilia; HR, intimal hemorrhage; ILI, intimal lymphocytic infiltration; IV, intimal vascularization; SDNP, sudden death without prodromata, SDP, sudden death with prodromata.

Table 8. Lymphocytic and plasma cell inflammatory reaction (IR) in coronary atherosclerotic plaques in different groups of population studied

	No. cases	IR%	No. stenoses	IR %	Mild	Moder	Severe
Acute infarct	100	100	491	75	34	21	20
Chronic IHD	50	88	175	74	32	13	29
Sudden death	208	83	1084	55	29	16	10
Healthy controls	97	64	371	41	22	14	5

Table 9. Lymphocytic and plasma cell inflammatory reaction (IR), proteoglycan accumulation (PA) and atheroma (AT) (expressed in percentage) related to intimal thickness and lumen reduction

Intimal thickness μm	IR	PA	AT	Lumen reduction %	IR	PA	AT
300	2	3	2	<50	32	52	27
600	28	50	16	50-69	62	70	54
1000	54	69	43	70-79	74	71	75
2000	73	75	69	80-89	84	71	77
>2000	79	57	76	>90	82	58	74

the inflammatory reaction was present in most, if not all stenoses, independent of its degree and the type of stenosis from the same patient. In controls it was absent or found only in one or a few stenoses. In ischemic heart disease groups, the inflammatory plaque reaction did not correlate with heart weight, extent of myocardial fibrosis or with old thrombus. It correlated with acute thrombus, infarct necrosis, coagulative myocytolysis and short severe stenoses. Furthermore, a significantly high frequency of this inflammation was observed in atherosclerotic plaques of the ascending aorta in sudden and unexpected death patients vscontrols. In AMI and chronic ischemic patient the aorta was not studied.

4. A prominent tropism of lymphocytic and plasma cell elements for adventitial nervous structures adjacent to the tunica media was noted.

No morphological variable demonstrated any change in respect to the age, gender, heart weight, extent of myocardial fibrosis or coronary medial thickness. Table 10 presents a synthesis of the main variations in characteristics of atherosclerotic plaques amongst our different clinical groups.

Table 10. Main significant variations of plaque variables in different groups

	AMI	CI	SDP	SDNP	AD
All stenoses	+ [a]	− [b]	+	ns[c]	−
Severe stenosis (≥70 %)	+	+	ns	ns	−
Concentric plaque	+	ns	−	ns	ns
Semilunar plaque	−	ns	+	ns	ns
Short stenoses (3 mm)	+	ns	ns	ns	+
Long stenoses (30 mm)	−	ns	ns	ns	ns
Intimal thickness ≥2000 µm	+	+	ns	ns	−
Intimal thickness ≤299 µm	−	−	−	−	+
Medial thickness ≥200 µm	ns	+	ns	ns	ns
Medial thickness ≤99 µm	+	ns	+	ns	ns
Atheroma or advential lymphocytic infiltrate or intimal lymphocytic infiltrate or calcification	+	+	ns	ns	−
Same variables in most stenoses in single case	+	+	ns	ns	−
Intimal hemorrhage	+	ns	−	−	−
Basophilia	+	−	ns	+	+
Intima vascularization	−	−	+	+	ns
Fibrosis plaque	−	−	+	−	+
Thrombosis					
Acute occlusive	+	ns	ns	ns	−
Acute mural	+	ns	ns	ns	−
Old occlusive	ns	+	ns	ns	−
Old mural	ns	ns	ns	ns	−

Abbreviations: AD, accidental death; AMI, acute myocardial infarction; CI, chronic ischemia; SDNP, sudden death without prodromata; SDP, sudden death with prodromata
[a] + in excess; [b] − in deficit.; [c] ns in expected range

Medial thickness and plaque variables

We found that maximal medial thickness ranged between 100 and 199 µm in the majority of vessel segments. It must be noted that medial changes were focally restricted to the region of atherosclerotic plaques only.

Medial thickness diminished significantly with both increasing intimal thickness and lumen reduction. This was particularly so with concentric plaques. The greatest medial thickness was associated with semilunar plaques and where lumen reduction was less than 70%. When maximal intimal and medial thickness were compared, irrespective of the degree of stenosis and type of plaque, both increased progressively until the intima was 2000 µm thick. With an intimal thickness greater than 2000 µm, there was an excess of both <99 and >200 µm widths of media. In semilunar stenoses the media in the normal part of the vessel wall tended to be thicker than at the plaque site. In concentric plaques medial width was mainly uniform at any site, circumferentially. Only occasionally were both media and intima of lesser thickness. In 34 sections (most in acute infarct cases) the media was focally absent with an associated intense lymphocytic and plasma cell inflammatory reaction. No relation was established between medial thickness and morphologic variables in a plaque.

Heart weight and plaque variables

A pathological heart weight ($\geq$500 g) was observed in 10% of control subjects; 43% of SD cases without extensive myocardial fibrosis; 76% of SD with extensive myocardial fibrosis; 39% of AMI without, and 53% associated with, extensive myocardial fibrosis (Table 11). The number of both mild and severe stenoses was significantly higher in heavy hearts when compared to normal ones. No relation was found between heart weight, gender, age and any other plaque variable.

Table 11. Maximal lumen reduction and number of vessels with severe stenosis ($\geq$70%) in relation to heart weight in different groups*

Heart weight (g)	Lumen reduction %		Total	Stenosis $\geq$70% in		
	<69	$\geq$70		1	2	3
					vessels	
AMI 1st						
<500	6	37	43	16	17	4
$\geq$500	4	23	27	13	6	4
Total	10	60	70	29	23	8
AMI 2nd						
<500	–	14	14	3	7	4
$\geq$500	1	15	16	6	6	3
Total	1	29	30	9	13	7
SD 1st						
<500	24	52	76	29	21	2
$\geq$500	22	35	57	11	13	11
Total	46	87	133	40	34	13
SD 2nd						
<500	2	16	18	3	6	7
$\geq$500	3	54	57	10	20	24
Total	5	70	75	13	26	31
AD						
<500	52	35	87	21	11	3
$\geq$500	7	3	10	1	2	–
Total	59	38	97	22	13	3

* In AMI the relation between heart weight and lumen reduction was calculated in 100 cases.

Coronary occlusion

In healthy controls only one acute mural thrombus was found in a coronary artery.

Amongst ischemic heart disease subjects the only type of acute occlusive lesion found in subepicardial coronary arteries and branches was a thrombus. Its frequency was 15% in 208 sudden death cases and 41% in 200 acute infarct patients. Acute mural thrombi figures were 10% and 18% respectively. An acute occlusive thrombus was observed significantly less frequently in sudden death cases but a significant excess of acute occlusive thrombi were seen in sudden death cases with extensive myocardial fibrosis (28%) and of acute mural thrombi in acute infarct cases without fibrosis (20%; Table 12). An old occlusive thrombus was present in 18% of AMI patients and in 6% of SD subjects. An old mural thrombus was seen in 4% of AMI and in 1% of SD cases.

In general, an acute occlusive thrombus was found in the infarct-related artery being located in the left anterior descending branch in 39, in the left circumflex branch in 11 and in the right coronary artery in 26 cases. In 6 cases more than 1 thrombus was found (LAD + RCA in 5, LCX + RCA in 1). The left anterior descending branch was the main infarct-related artery in 52% of cases, the right coronary artery in 36% and the left circumflex branch in 11%.

We found the majority of these occlusive and mural thrombi in an area of severe ($\geq$70%) luminal stenosis, that lesion being mainly concentric and longer than 3 mm. These acute thrombi were significantly associated with advential/intimal inflammation, intimal hemorrhage, atheroma and calcification in the plaque. In contrast, old organized thrombi were related to a significant absence of morphologic plaque variables and associated with fibrous plaques.

Table 12. Frequency of acute occlusive and mural thrombi in acute infarcts and sudden coronary deaths

Source	Total	(%)	Thrombus			
			occlusive		mural	
AMI 1st	145	(100)	60	(41)	29	(20)
AMI 2nd	55	(100)	22	(40)*	7	(13)
Total	200	(100)	82	(41)	36	(18)
SD 1st	133	(100)	11	(8)	14	(10)
SD 2nd	75	(100)	21	(28)	8	(11)
Total	208	(100)	32	(15)	22	(10)

*An occlusive thrombus was not in the supplying artery in one patient (not included).
In control group only one mural thrombus found.

Amongst AMI cases acute occlusive thrombi increased in frequency statistically with an increasing infarct size, (see below); a behavior not shown by mural thrombi (Table 13).

INTRAMURAL VASCULAR LESIONS

No heart in any of our studies, even in the presence of severe atherosclerosis of extramural arteries, showed an atherosclerotic plaque in an intramural arterial vessel.

Table 13. Percentage distribution of acute coronary thrombus in 200 acute infarcts (AMI) and 208 sudden coronary death (SD) in relation to atherosclerotic plaque variables, infarct size and survival

	AMI thrombus		SD thrombus	
	occlusive	mural	occlusive	mural
Total	41	18	15	11
ATS plaque stenosis %				
≤69	7	14	–	9
70-79	33	36	16	20
80-89	35	19	47	45
>90	24	31	38	32
Length mm				
≤5	6	19	6	9
5-20	38	39	19	27
>20	56	42	75	64
Type				
concentric	100	100	94	91
atheromatous	84	81	75	82
Lymph-plasm inflam.	92	82	92	79
Infarct size %				
≤10	20	17	–	–
11-20	32	19	–	–
21-30	48	33	–	–
31-40	44	19	–	–
41-50	78	8	–	–
>50	86	3	–	–
Survival days AMI				
≤2	29	–	–	–
3-10	51	–	–	–
11-30	45	–	–	–
Survival minutes SD				
<10	–	–	12	–
10-60	–	–	23	–
61-180	–	–	30	–

Fibrous thickening of the intima

The different types of intimal thickening described in subepicardial arterial vessels (see chapter 3) were never seen in intramural arterial branches. In general, a fibrous intimal thickening affected small arteries surrounding or within scar tissue or adjacent to the annulus fibrosis or the membranous interventricular septum. This occurred without any difference in frequency between groups of subjects. In particular, intimal thickening of the arterial branch to the sinus node was present in 2% of SD and AD cases and in 10% and 14% of these cases respectively in the arterial branch of the A-V node.

Subintimal hyaline material

This was observed as small nodular deposits in people older than 50 years. Only one or occasionally a few intramural arterial vessels (maximum 14 in a SD case) were involved. Exceptionally, this deposit appeared to stenose the lumen, the reduction being generally semilunar, and not exceeding 50%. Its exact nature was not determined (negative stain for amyloid).

Perivascular fibrosis

Perivascular fibrosis of intramural arterial vessels was another rare finding in the absence of myocardial fibrosis.

Atheromatous emboli

In more than 14,000 myocardial sections of all groups only one *atheromatous* embolus, associated with reactive intimal proliferation, was observed in an interventricular septal arterial branch. The adjacent myocardium was normal. The subject was a SD case who had one severe atherosclerotic stenosis of the anterior descending coronary branch and ulcerated atherosclerotic plaques of the aorta.

Occlusive arterial platelet aggregates

Platelet aggregates could be demonstrated in the heart of SD cases as frequently as in controls (70% vs 76%) but they were infrequent in either sample (Table 14). No pathological changes of the vessel wall were noted associated with them.

A significant relationship was found between the frequency of arterial platelet aggregates—particularly in the AD subjects (P <0.05 for trend)—and a longer interval from onset of terminal episode to death (Table 15).

No relation was observed between the presence of occlusive and mural thrombi in extramural coronary arteries or the presence of demonstrable infarct necrosis and Zenker necrosis and the frequency of arterial platelet aggregates. The relationship between the degree of lumen reduction, the frequency of cases and the number of intramural arterial vessels with platelet aggregates did not show any significant

Table 14. Frequency of platelet aggregates and number of occluded intramural arterial vessels in sudden death (SD) and control (AD) cases

Total cases	SD	(%)	AD	(%)
Arterial platelet aggregates	208	(100)	97	(100)
absent	61	(29)	23	(24)
present in	147	(71)	74	(76)
<5	77	(37)	35	(36)
5 - 10	37	(18)	14	(14)
11-20	22	(10)	11	(11)
21-30	7	(3)	5	(5)
31-60	4	(2)	9	(9)
vessels				
Total sections	3328	(100)	1552	(100)
absent	2793	(84)	1273	(82)
present in	535	(16)	279	(18)
1	269	(8)	124	(8)
2	134	(4)	62	(4)
3	61	(2)	40	(3)
4	26	(1)	21	(1)
5-15	45	(1)	32	(2)
vessels				

Table 15. Frequency of arterial platelet aggregates versus survival time

Survival Time (min)	Total cases (%)	Platelet aggregates				
		absent	present	<5	5-10	≥10 vessels
SD						
<10	151 (100)	51 (34)	100 (66)	52 (34)	26 (17)	22 (14)
≥10	57 (100)	10 (17)	47 (82)	25 (44)	11 (19)	11 (19)
AD						
<10	75 (100)	22 (29)	53 (71)	30 (40)	11 (15)	12 (16)
≥10	22 (100)	1 (5)	21 (95)	5 (23)	3 (14)	13 (59)

divergence between AD and SD groups. Finally, platelet aggregates were rarely observed within the conduction system being present in one instance in the sinus node of one SD case, and in the A-V node—His bundle of five SD and four AD cases.

Blood stasis versus platelet aggregates:

Blood stasis (see method) was *not* demonstrated in 30% of total sections from the sudden death group and 40% of the AD group. Associated arterial and venous intramural stasis was seen in 45% and 40%, while venous intramural stasis alone was present in 24% and

19% respectively (Table 16). Arterial and venous intramural stasis was significantly more frequent (P<0.001) in the SED group. In both SD and AD cases, where stasis was present, a single line of red blood cells or polymorphonuclear leukocytes or platelet aggregates were frequently seen layered in the vessels. The separation of blood elements was particularly evident in longitudinal sections of arterioles, the proximal tract being filled by red cells and the distal by granular material. Furthermore, adjacent cross sectioned vessels, likely branches of the same stem, showed all possible combinations of these findings.

The frequency of both arterial and venous platelet aggregates directly correlated with the presence and type of intramural blood stasis in all groups (Table 16). In the case of venous stasis alone, only venous platelet aggregates showed a maximal frequency.

Medial hyperplasia obliterans

Medial hyperplasia obliterans was found in 58% of SUD, 46% of SED and in 78% of AD cases (Table 17). The higher frequency in the latter is statistically significant. The distribution of medial hyperplasia was greatest in papillary muscles, columnae carneae and the interventricular septum in all groups. A higher frequency of this vascular change was observed in the anterior papillary muscle than in the posterior one of either ventricle. No relationship was found with either a patient's gender or age. The frequency was practically the same in different decades of all subjects (Table 18). No relationship between myocardial fibrosis and medial hyperplasia was observed nor between intramural medial hyperplasia and atherosclerotic obstructive damage of the subepicardial coronary arteries or heart weight.

Table 16. Frequency of arterial (AP) and venous (VP) platelet aggregates in relation to intramural blood stasis (total sections), in sudden unexpected death (SD) and control cases (AD)

	SD (%)	AD (%)
No demonstrable stasis	1005 (100)	629 (100)
+ AP	60 (6)	48 (8)
+VP	29 (3)	5 (1)
Arterial + venous stasis	1512 (100)	620 (100)
+ AP	454 (30)	217 (35)
+VP	418 (28)	210 (34)
Venous stasis alone	811 (100)	303 (100)
+AP	21 (3)	14 (5)
+VP	283 (35)	107 (35)
Total sections	3328 (100)	1552 (100)
+ AP	535 (16)	279 (18)
+ VP	730 (22)	322 (21)

Table 17. Frequency distribution of medial hyperplasia obliterans (MH) and its location

			Location							Number of locations				
Total	Cases (%)	Cases + MH	LV	LPM	RV	RPM	IS	A	CS	1	2	3	4	5
SD	208 (100)	109 (52)	12	73	7	21	46	4	3	66	30	12	1	–
AD	97 (100)	76 (78)	10	56	5	22	36	–	–	39	26	8	1	2

LV, RV left and right ventricles; LPM, RPM left and right papillary muscles; IS interventricular septum; A atria; CS conduction system

Table 18. Medial hyperplasia obliterans in relation to age and sex

	SD				AD			
Decade	M	F	Tot. (%)*	Total cases	M	F	Tot. (%)*	Total cases
<40	13	2	15 (43)	35	6	1	7 (70)	10
40-49	16	2	18 (54)	33	7	2	9 (69)	13
50-59	33	2	35 (51)	68	24	–	24 (86)	28
60-69	21	3	24 (53)	45	14	3	18 (78)	23
>70	11	6	17 (63)	27	17	1	18 (78)	23
Total	94	15	109 (52)	208	69	7	76 (78)	97

* Percentage of total cases per decade

MORPHOLOGY OF MYOCARDIAL DAMAGE

Acute myocardial infarction

There was a myocardial infarct of different size in all 200 AMI cases included in our study. (See chapter 3 for definition of myocardial infarction.)

Location

The infarct had an anterior or anteroseptal location in the left ventricle in 39% of cases, was posterior or posteroseptal in 28% and anteroposterior in 32%. It involved the luminal third of the left ventricular wall in 23 patients (2 with occlusive thrombus), the inner two-thirds of the wall in 62 patients (26 with occlusive thrombus) and was transmural in 115 (54 with occlusive thrombus; Table 19).

Size

Overall, infarcts ranged from less than 10% of left ventricular mass to more than 50%, with the maximum being 85%. About half of all 200 fatal infarcts were of a small size (less than 20% of left ventricular mass). Infarct size had a different distribution when acute infarctions that occurred in apparently healthy people (*1st episode*) were compared with those that occurred in patients with known IHD (*2nd episode*)

(Table 20). In particular, *2nd episode* infarcts showed a size less than 10% in half and less than 20% in 64% of cases. In AMI *1st episode* the figures were 22% and 43% respectively.

Relationship to coronary artery lesions

The frequency of acute occlusive and mural thrombi related to infarct size is reported in Table 21. A significant correlation exists between the occurrence of acute occlusive thrombi and infarct size. In infarcts smaller than 10% of left ventricular mass their frequency was 20%, increasing progressively to a maximum of 86% with an infarct size of >50%. Their occurrence in men (46%) was not significantly more frequent than in women (31%).

Infarct size did not correlate with the number, (Table 22) or degree and length (Table 23) of severe stenoses present in the whole coronary arterial system.

Survival

When the survival time of all 200 AMI patients was considered (Table 24), of those with small infarcts (≤20% of left ventricular mass) 64% had a short survival period (<2 days). In contrast, of those with large infarcts half survived more than 11 days. These findings (P <0.01)

Table 19. Relationship of infarct size (% left ventricular mass), location in the left ventricular wall and acute occlusive thrombus in supplying artery

Location	Infarct size (%)												
	≤10		11-20		21-30		31-40		41-50		>50		Total	
	P	T	P	T	P	T	P	T	P	T	P	T	P	T
Inner 1/3	22	2	1	1*	–	–	–	–	–	–	–	–	23	2
Inner 2/3	22	6	18	7	14	7	4	2	1	1	3	3	62	26
Transmural	16	4	18	4	30	14	23	10	17	13	11	9	115	54
Total	60	12	37	11	44	21	27	12	18	14	14	12	200	82

P = patients; T = thrombi
* An occlusive thrombus not in supplying artery in one patient (not included).

Table 20. Distribution of infarct size (% left ventricular mass) in 200 consecutive acute infarct cases without (AMI 1st episode) and with (AMI 2nd episode) extensive myocardial fibrosis

Source	Cases (%)	Infarct size (%)					
		≤10	11-20	21-30	31-40	41-50	>50
AMI 1st	145 (100)	32 (22)	30 (21)	32 (22)	24 (16)	14 (10)	13 (9)
AMI 2nd	55 (100)	28 (51)	7 (13)	12 (22)	3 (5)	4 (7)	1 (2)
Total	200 (100)	60 (30)	37 (19)	44 (22)	27 (13)	18 (9)	14 (7)

were similar in both *1st* and *2nd episode* patients, who also showed no significant divergency in age and gender distribution.

No relationship could be established between survival, infarct size and the frequency of an acute occlusive thrombus (Table 25). In Table 26 infarct size is related to the main supplying artery or branch. The left

Table 21. Infarct size, (% left ventricular mass) maximal lumen reduction and frequency of thrombus in supplying artery

| Infarct size % | Cases | Luminal Stenosis (%) | | | | | | | | | | | | | | |
| | | ≤59 | | | 60-69 | | | 70-79 | | | 80-89 | | | ≥90 | | |
		N	O	M	N	O	M	N	O	M	N	O	M	N	O	M
≤10	60	3	1	1	5	–	–	10	1	2	8	7	–	16	3	3
11-20	37	4	–	–	1	–	–	5	6	3	4	3	–	4	3	4
21-30	44	2	–	–	1	–	2	2	7	3	3	7	4	3	7	3
31-40	27	3	–	–	1	1	1	3	5	3	2	3	2	–	2	1
41-50	18	–	–	–	–	–	1	–	3	1	1	7	1	–	4	–
>50	14	–	3	–	–	1	–	–	5	1	–	2	–	1	1	–
Total	200	12	4	1	8	2	4	20	27	13	18	29	7	24	20	11

N = no thrombus; O = occlusive thrombus; M = mural thrombus

Table 22. Lack of relationship between number of severe coronary artery stenoses (≥70%) and infarct size (% left ventricular mass) in 200 consecutive acute infarct cases

| Infarct size (%) | Lumen reduction (%) | | | | | |
	<69	≥70	in 1	2	3 vessel	Total (%)
≤20	7 (7)	90 (93)	39 (40)	37 (38)	14 (14)	97 (100)
>20	10 (10)	93 (90)	38 (37)	34 (33)	21 (20)	103 (100)
Total	17 (8)	183 (91)	77 (38)	71 (35)	35 (17)	200 (100)

P < 0.05 for trend

Table 23. Degree and length of maximal stenosis in supplying artery related to presence of acute thrombus in acute infarcts

| Luminal stenosis (%) | Length stenosis (mm) | | | |
	<5	5-20	>20	Total
<69				
Occlusive thrombus	1	2	3	6
Mural thrombus	1	3	1	5
No thrombus	12	6	2	20
≥70				
Occlusive thrombus	7	26	43	76
Mural thrombus	6	11	14	31
No thrombus	28	19	15	62

Table 24. Distribution of infarct size (% left ventricular mass) versus survival in 200 consecutive acute infarct cases

Survival days	Cases (%)	Infarct size (%)					
		<10	11-20	21-30	31-40	41-50	>50
<2	70 (100)	34 (48)	11 (16)	11 (16)	9 (13)	1 (1)	4 (6)
3-10	74 (100)	17 (23)	9 (12)	24 (32)	10 (14)	9 (12)	5 (7)
11-30	56 (100)	9 (16)	17 (31)	9 (16)	8 (14)	8 (14)	5 (9)
Total	200 (100)	60 (30)	37 (18)	44 (22)	27 (14)	18 (9)	14 (7)

Table 25. Infarct size (% left ventricular mass), survival time and acute occlusive coronary thrombus

Survival days	Infarct size (%)												
	≤10		11-20		21-30		31-40		41-50		>50		Total	
	P	T	P	T	P	T	P	T	P	T	P	T	P	T
≤2	34	6	11	2	11	4	9	4	1	1	4	3	70	20
3-10	17	2	9	4	24	14	10	6	9	8	5	4	74	38
≥11	9	4	17	5	9	3	8	2	8	5	5	5	56	24
Total	60	12	37	11*	44	21	27	12	18	14	14	12	200	82

P = patients; T = thrombi
* Occlusive thrombus not in supplying artery in one patient.

Table 26. Infarct size (% left ventricular mass) in relation to its main supplying vessel

Vessel	Infarct size %						
	≤10	11-20	21-30	31-40	41-50	>50	Total (%)
Left anterior descending	33 (31)	17 (16)	20 (19)	12 (11)	12 (11)	11 (10)	105 (100)
Left circumflex	8 (35)	5 (22)	6 (26)	3 (13)	–	1 (4)	23 (100)
Right coronary artery	19 (26)	15 (21)	18 (25)	12 (17)	6 (8)	2 (3)	72 (100)
Total	60 (30)	37 (18)	44 (22)	27 (13)	18 (9)	14 (7)	200 (100)

anterior descending branch usually supplied the largest infarcts. It must be noted that in 37% of our cases, an infarct involved the adjacent vascular territories of vessels that were not demonstrably occluded. No difference could be demonstrated between men and women with respect to survival time and the size of the infarct they developed; nor between survival time and heart weight or between heart weight and infarct size. Despite a similar distribution of pathologic heart weight (≥500 g) in different decades of life, hypertrophy of the heart generally was significantly more frequent in men (69%) than in women (39%) in this AMI group.

Other forms of myocardial necrosis associated with infarction

All AMI cases showed in continuity with the peripheral layer of infarct necrosis, (but not in subendocardial or perivascular myocardium), multifocal or extensive confluent areas of *Zenker necrosis* of varying size. Furthermore, most hearts (85%) had in the normal myocardium in the vicinity of the infarct as well as in other areas of myocardium far removed from the infarct, isolated or sometime confluent foci of this type of necrosis. The presence of this lesion could not be correlated with the degree of coronary damage, the size of an infarct or the presence or absence of an acute occlusive thrombus.

In 38% of infarcted hearts, *colliquative myocytolysis* was observed in the subendocardial and perivascular myocardium within or adjacent to the infarct. The presence of this lesion too, did not correlate with the degree of coronary damage, the size of an infarct or the presence or absence of an acute occlusive thrombus. About half of these hearts also showed extensive fibrosis in adjacent myocardium. (See chapter 3 for definition of these forms of myocardial necrosis.)

Association of different forms of myocardial necrosis and fibrosis in sudden coronary death

Myocardial necrosis

The different types of myocardial necrosis and the extent of fibrosis found in relation to the degree of coronary artery lumen narrowing and the presence of acute occlusive thrombi in SD cases are presented in Table 27.

An *acute infarct* was documented histologically in only 17% of 208 sudden death cases, in 12% of 106 SUD and 25% of 102 SED cases. The area of necrosis was large in 8, (>20% of left ventricular mass), small (≤20%) in 16 and microfocal in 11 cases. The occurrence and extent of an infarct did not correlate with the degree and number of severe coronary artery stenoses. An acute occlusive thrombus was detected in a subtending vessel in 50% of 16 SUD cases and 16% of 19 SED cases. All but two instances had the thrombus in an area of severe coronary stenosis. According to its histologic pattern the infarct was judged at an early stage (6-12 hrs) in 7 cases of each group, while it was older than one day in the remainder. In most cases infarct necrosis was associated with old myocardial fibrosis, particularly in SED cases.

Zenker necrosis was the most frequent form of myocardial necrosis found in SD cases. It was observed as the only acute lesion in 72% of these individuals and in 20% of AD cases. In all but three of the latter the lesion was minimal while in SD hearts it was moderately extensive in 29%. In most AD subjects and in about two-third of the SD cases this type of necrosis was *early*; whereas in 13% of SD and 4% of AD cases it was *alveolar;* a *healing stage* was seen in 12% and

Table 27. Type of myocardial necrosis and fibrosis, lumen reduction and acute occlusive thrombus in sudden death cases

Myocardial damage	Lumen reduction % <69	Lumen reduction % ≥70	Total	≥70% in 1	≥70% in 2 vessels	≥70% in 3	Acute occl. thr.
Infarct							
≤10	–	11	11	3	4	4	1
11-30	–	16	16	4	8	4	6
>30	2	6	8	5	1	–	4
Total	2	33	35	12	13	8	11
Zenker necrosis							
Minimal	23	65	88	16	25	24	7
Moderate	6	32	38	8	14	10	9
Extensive	5	18	23	8	9	1	9
Total	34	115	149	32	48	35	25
Early	27	68	95	21	25	22	9
Alveolar	1	27	28	7	9	11	9
Scarring	6	20	26	4	14	2	7
Total	34	115	149	32	48	35	25
Myocytolysis							
Minimal	–	16	16	1	5	10	2
Fibrosis							
No or minimal	39	64	103	32	24	8	15
Moderate	4	44	48	13	15	16	4
Extensive	1	56	57	12	15	29	5
Total	44	164	208	57	54	53	24

1% respectively. Among 28 SD cases with normal coronary arteries or a lumen reduction less than 50%, Zenker necrosis was observed in 78% of cases. In all 35 SD cases with infarct necrosis, Zenker necrosis was seen at the perimeter of the infarct and in 83% elsewhere in normal myocardium. No relationship was demonstrated between its presence and the extent and degree of coronary obstruction or the presence or absence of an occlusive coronary thrombus.

Minimal foci of subendocardial *colliquative myocytolysis* were observed in only 8% of 208 SD cases. All but two examples were in SED subjects with both pathological heart weights (≥500 g) and extensive old myocardial fibrosis.

Myocardial fibrosis

In general AD subjects showed minimal fibrosis. In only 5% of cases was a single, small focus visible grossly. In contrast, fibrosis was moderate (<10%) in 12% and extensive (≥10%)in 10% of the SUD group and 32% and 18% respectively amongst the SED group. Conversely, in SUD and SED cases, moderate and extensive fibrosis tended to significantly increase with an increasing number of coronary vessels that showed severe stenoses. Recent myocardial fibrosis was seen in 31 SD cases. It was isolated in 5, associated with old fibrosis in 16 and old fibrosis plus infarct necrosis in 10, the lesion being located in different areas. Most foci were minimal, only two being extensive and two median. In general, no correlation was found between the frequency of thrombus, incidence/extension of acute necroses and myocardial fibrosis and increasing heart weight.

The different patterns of acute irreversible myocardial damage and fibrosis were seen more frequently in the left ventricular free wall, followed by the interventricular septum and then the right ventricle. Acute irreversible damage was not seen in the conduction system and only in 8 SUD and 10 SED cases were microfoci of old myocardial fibrosis observed. No relationship was found between survival time, activity and the degree of coronary obstructive damage, type and extension of myocardial necrosis or heart weight (Table 28).

Table 28. Survival, activity and symptoms before sudden death in relation to coronary and myocardial damage and heart weight

	Total cases	≤69%	≥70% in 1	2	≥3 Vessels	Ac. occl. thrombus	Acute Infarct	Zenker necrosis	Fibrosis	Heart weight ≥500 g
Survival										
<10 min.	151	41	39	41	30	18	25	110	123	68
10-60 min.	47	9	11	17	10	11	8	33	37	18
>60 min.	10	1	3	2	4	3	2	6	10	1
Total	208	51	53	60	44	32	35	149	170	87
Activity										
Working	52	10	22	11	9	5	6	37	40	22
Walking	44	7	11	13	13	5	7	37	40	17
Driving	13	–	1	9	3	1	2	9	12	5
Sleeping	22	9	5	5	3	4	5	13	20	9
Resting	72	23	12	21	16	17	14	51	56	33
Unknown	5	2	2	1	-	–	1	2	2	1
Total	208	51	53	60	44	32	35	149	170	87
Symptoms										
Angina	48	4	20	12	12	11	9	32	35	16
Dyspnea	29	12	6	8	3	3	6	24	25	14
Paresthesia	3	–	1	2	-	2	1	3	3	–
Vertigo	4	–	1	3	-	–	1	4	4	2
Unknown	124	35	25	35	29	16	18	86	103	55
Total	208	51	53	60	44	32	35	149	170	87

A comparison between 102 subjects with (SED), and 106 without (SUD), prodromata showed a statistically significant higher frequency of acute occlusive thrombi in the SUD group while in the SED group a coronary stenosis greater than 90%, triple severe stenoses (≥70%), extensive myocardial fibrosis, demonstrable acute infarct and a pathological heart weight (≥500 g) prevailed.

Heart rupture

AMI cases

Among 200 acute infarct cases 27 died of cardiac tamponade following rupture of the left ventricular free wall at the site of transmural infarct necrosis. In 2 other cases the rupture was located in the interventricular septum and in another 5 the left anterior (2) or posterior (3) papillary muscle had ruptured.

The majority (31) of these ruptures occurred in *1st episode* AMI cases (Table 29). A significantly higher frequency of rupture was observed in hearts with an infarct size of 21-30% of left ventricular mass (30%), followed by an infarct size of 11-20% (27%). In only three *2nd episode* cases was a rupture present. The percentage distribution was 21% for the *1st episode* cases versus 5% for the *2nd episode* cases. This difference was significant. The frequency of an occlusive thrombus was 50% in the 34 hearts that had ruptured compared to 40% in 166 hearts that had not. However, this difference was not statistically significant. No relation was found between the degree and number of coronary stenoses or heart weight and rupture of the heart.

Table 29. Heart rupture as a cause of death in 200 consecutive acute myocardial infarcts

Source	No	Infarct size % (% left ventricular mass)						Lumen reduction %					Occlusive thrombus
		<10	11-20	21-30	31-40	41-50	>50	<69	≥70	1	2	3 vess.	
AMI 1st													
+ rpt	31	2	10	11	3	3	2	3	28	15	9	4	15
no	114	30	20	21	21	11	11	13	101	46	40	15	45
Total	145	32	30	32	24	14	13	16	129	61	49	19	60
AMI 2nd													
+ rpt	3	1	–	2	–	–	–	–	3	2	1	–	2
no	52	27	7	10	3	4	1	1	51	14	21	16	20
Total	55	28	7	12	3	4	1	1	54	16	22	16	22
Grand Total	200	60	37	44	27	18	14	17	183	77	71	35	82
+ rpt	34	3	10	13	3	3	2	3	31	17	10	4	17

1st, first episode of IHD; 2nd, chronic IHD; rpt, rupture of the heart

SD cases

Amongst 208 sudden and unexpected death cases only 1 had ruptured the left anterior free wall. The small rupture, without associated cardiac tamponade, occurred in a zone with extensive, confluent, Zenker necrosis. Not 1 of the 35 acute infarcts documented amongst these cases was associated with a cardiac rupture.

PERTINENT FINDINGS
FROM OTHER PERSONAL STUDIES

PLASTIC CASTS OF CORONARY VESSELS: COLLATERALS

Plastic casts of the coronary arteries in normal human hearts demonstrate an extensive network of both homo- and intercoronary anastomoses, or collaterals, in all cardiac regions. The collaterals join adjacent arterial vessels at different levels along their course and within the whole thickness of the cardiac wall. They have a characteristic finely coiled appearance which seems related to their course, parallel to the line of cardiac muscle contraction.

Human collateral vessels are intramural in location. In normal hearts they have a capillary-like wall. However, two hearts, one normal and one associated with severe coronary artery stenoses, showed respectively one capillary-like superficial collateral 100 μm in diameter, or large anatomoses 500-1000 μm or more in diameter, in the interstitial tissue between visceral pericardium and myocardium. The latter vessels had a very thin media with a fragmented and ill-defined intimal elastic lamina. The diameter of collaterals in normal hearts range from less than 20 to 350 μm with an anastomotic index (see above) ranging from 3 to 6 (mean 5). In atrophic hearts with normal coronary arteries the index was 2 to 6 (mean 4); amongst hypertrophied hearts with normal coronary arteries the figures were 4 to 14 (mean 7). Normal hearts from subjects with chronic anemia had an index of 9 to 19 (mean 12).

In the presence of atherosclerotic stenosis with a lumen/diameter reduction greater than 70% the diameter and length of collaterals increased dramatically so that they might exceed 1000 μm in diameter and several centimeters in length. Any severely obstructive coronary artery lesion, even multiple ones, was/were always found associated with enlarged collaterals. These could be intercoronary or homocoronary vessels that bypassed the obstruction(s) (satellite anastomoses). Often, a peculiar *plaque satellite anastomotic network* was seen at the site of a severe luminal stenosis. It consisted of a mesh of channels which joined small branches of the parent vessel proximal and distal to the obstruction. The anastomotic index in these instances ranged from 5 to 33 with a mean value of 16 associated with a single stenosis and of 22 in multiple severe stenoses. The presence or absence of a myocardial infarct was independent of the number of enlarged collaterals. In other words, hearts with the same degree of obstructive coronary damage could show a similar pattern of collateral enlargement not related to their myocardial status, whether normal or affected by an acute infarction or fibrosis of any extent. In particular, SD cases did not show any divergency in respect to the number and size of collaterals. According to the anastomotic index collateral enlargement increased proportionally with an increasing degree of stenosis and the number of severely obstructed coronary vessels in each heart.

CHRONOLOGICAL RELATIONSHIP
BETWEEN OCCLUSIVE THROMBUS AND INFARCT NECROSIS

Studying the chronological relationship between occlusive thrombi and infarct necrosis, an occlusive thrombus was present in 47% of the 208 AMI patients with a possible coeval correlation with the age of myocardial infarct in 48, in 47% of the 54 unexpected SD subjects, with a chronological correlation in 25 and in 46% of the 57 expected SD individuals with correlation in 23. The thrombus occluded a small residual lumen at the site of a critical stenosis induced by an atherosclerotic plaque in most AMI and SD cases and was often associated with an advential and intimal inflammatory reaction.

PLATELET AGGREGATES AND MICROANGIOPATHY
IN THROMBOTIC THROMBOCYTOPENIC PURPURA

Of 39 TTP cases examined, 90% died within 35 days of the onset of symptoms: survival time ranged from 4 to 300 days (average 37). In these cases typical clinical findings were: (1) hemorrhagic (87%); (2) neurologic (84%); (3) mental disorders (76%); (4) severe hemolytic anemia (97%) (in 70% of cases there was less than 2.5 million red cells and 50% hemoglobin) and (5) thrombocytopenia (99% less than 80,000 platelets/mm^3 50% less than 50,000 platelets/mm^3). In no instance did a patient have angina pectoris or clinical evidence of a myocardial infarction. Only 2 cases with manifest and typical TTP clinical symptoms lasting more than 5 days, died suddenly in hospital. Generally, death occurred after prolonged coma or shock (61%) or convulsions with neurologic symptoms (33%).

The pathognomic stenosing microangiopathy was evident and severe in the myocardium. Often, most intramural arterioles in a histological section seemed occluded or severely stenosed by PAS-positive material. The latter appeared covered by normal endothelium. Superimposed on this hyaline glycoprotein material, platelet aggregates were demonstrated, particularly by serial sections. Occlusion of normal arterioles by platelet aggregates was also a usual finding. In all cases the myocardium was normal, except for a few microscopic foci of Zenker necrosis in 31% of cases and hemorrhage in 79%. No spatial relationship could be demonstrated between the microangiopathy and myocardial damage in serial sections.

RED BLOOD CELL PLUGGING IN SICKLE CELL ANEMIA

Microcirculatory impairment occurs in sickle cell anemia with typical sickle red cell "plugging" particularly in the terminal arterial bed. In the 53 patients studied and despite histological documentation of diffuse sickle cell aggregation, no clinical or pathological findings of ischemic heart disease were found.

CHAPTER 2

SUDDEN CORONARY DEATH— FINDINGS IN THE LITERATURE

Any reviewer of the literature on sudden death faces different criteria of selection, dissimilar methods of examination and divergent definitions making exact comparison of data difficult. For instance, in several studies only cases with at least one coronary stenosis greater than 50% of lumen diameter or 75% of luminal area were included. At first glance such selection seems correct in relation to the postulate that sudden death can be *coronary* only in the presence of a functionally obstructive lesion. However, this postulate which will be discussed later, is still controversial and this type of selection in pathologic studies may bias conclusions. The general impression is a lack of discrimination in these studies between morphologic findings linked with sudden death and those that might be related to (a) chronic aspects of ischemic heart disease (*unexpected* versus *expected*); or (b) acute complications, e.g., coronary thrombus, etc. which may not be responsible for death; or (c) medical procedures such as prolonged therapy and/or resuscitation (*iatrogenic changes*). A similar lack of discrimination exists between *initial* and *terminal* morphologic features in relation to *survival time*. Finally, the frequent lack of control subjects, e.g., accidental death or noncardiac patients in such studies makes unpredictable the pathogenic significance of any lesion found.

With these reservations in mind, we collated from the literature the main pathological reports related to sudden coronary death. In presenting them we have been selective because some data may not have been given in reviewed papers. We avoid any comment with respect to our personal findings quoted above in the tables. The aim is to present the reader facts (or fictions?) which allow argument and offer an objective prelude to a review of the natural history (chapter 3) and functional significance (chapter 4) of pathological changes considered the core of various pathogenic hypotheses in ischemic heart disease (chapter 5).

GENDER AND AGE DISTRIBUTION

Amongst 23 studies (Table 30) the man to woman ratio (M/W) ranged from 1 to 16 (mean 6 ± 4). In four reports, where both whites and blacks were considered, the prevalence amongst males was less in blacks. The mean age per gender was referred to in only 5 of the 23 papers. In all but one the mean age of women who died suddenly, was higher (W 63 ± 6, M 58 ± 4 years).

CORONARY ATHEROSCLEROSIS

Frequently, amongst reviewed reports, the degree of coronary artery lumen reduction was not cited or was calculated using methods that are difficult to compare.

Table 30. Sex and age distribution in sudden coronary death. Reports in the literature.

Source	Year		Total cases	M	W	M/W ratio	Mean Age M	W
Bedford	1933		63	57	6	9	61	56
Levy	1936		24	21	3	7	–	–
Munck	1946		396	334	62	5	55	63
Rabson	1948		617	581	36	16	–	–
Croce	1960		824	719	105	7	–	–
Adelson	1961	W	433	389	44	9	–	–
		B	67	53	14	4		
Franco	1962		187	110	77	1	–	–
Spiekerman	1962		94	73	21	3	–	–
Jorgensen	1968		38	26	12	2	60	65
Luke	1968	W	59	55	4	14		
		B	19	15	4	4		
Scott	1972	W	175	145	30	5	59	
		B	13	8	5	2		
Titus	1970		86	65	21	3	60	
Friedman	1973		64	58	6	10	53	
Liberthson	1974		220	191	29	7	53	60
Lie	1975		406	298	108	3	59	
Haerem	1975		47	33	14	2	62	72
Margolis	1975		29	27	2	13	54	
Perper	1975	W	109	85	24	3	–	–
		B	60	48	12	4	–	–
Reichenbach	1977		87	78	9	9	63	
Warnes	1984		70	63	7	9	–	–
Falk	1984		25	20	5	4	–	–
Arbustini	1991		27	20	7	3	–	–
Lie	1991		202	157	45	3	–	–
Mean			164	138	26	6	–	–
SD			201.9	178.8	29.9	4	–	–
Personal	1979		208	182	26	7	53	56

We preferred to distinguish *functional* and *nonfunctional* stenoses according to the definition given in papers when such a distinction was clearly outlined. From 9 papers the number of SD cases with mild, nonfunctional stenosis in the whole coronary arterial system was 269 (16%) of the total 1648 cases (Table 31).

ACUTE CORONARY THROMBOSIS

In the literature the finding of an associated occlusive coronary artery thrombus in pathology papers ranged from 4% in cases with "instantaneous" death to 82% in sudden death with a survival of 24 hours (Friedman et al, 1973). The average frequency of an occlusive coronary thrombus amongst 4,524 cases of sudden coronary death reported in Table 32 was 29%. In the 27 papers cited in Table 32, only 4 mentioned the frequency of mural thrombi (Crawford et al, 1961; Newman et al, 1982; Warnes et al, 1984; Davies et al, 1984). Amongst those 310 cases 22% had mural (or intraluminal/intraintimal after Davies) thrombi. Their frequency in these studies ranged from 3% to 35%. There is agreement in pathological studies that the occlusive coronary thrombus is generally located at a site of a severe "functional" luminal stenosis (Baba et al, 1975; Warnes et al, 1984; Davies et al, 1984).

The frequency of plaque rupture was mentioned in 8 studies as follows: 12% amongst 75 cases (Crawford et al, 1961); 54%, 5 associated with thrombus (Friedman et al, 1973); 5% (Liberthson et al, 1975);

Table 31. Atherosclerotic lumen reduction and sudden coronary death. Reports in the literature.

Source	Year	Total cases	Functional stenosis No (%)	Functional stenosis Yes (%)	Functional stenosis in 1	Functional stenosis in 2 vess.	Functional stenosis in 3
Moritz	1946	115	31 (27)	84 (73)	–	–	–
Adelson	1961	500	162 (32)	338 (68)	–	–	–
Friedman	1973	59	4 (7)	55 (93)	9 (15)	11 (19)	35 (59)
Liberthson	1974	220	13 (6)	207 (94)	29 (13)	54 (25)	24 (56)
Lie	1975	406	29 (7)	377 (93)	–	–	–
Perper	1975	169	16 (9)	153 (91)	25 (15)	25 (15)	103 (61)
Reichenbach	1977	87	7 (8)	80 (92)	7 (8)	16 (18)	57 (66)
Newman	1982	65	5 (8)	60 (92)	11 (17)	17 (26)	32 (49)
Arbustini	1991	27	2 (7)	25 (93)	3 (11)	7 (26)	15 (56)
Total		1648 (100)	269 (16)	1379 (84)	84 (13)	130 (21)	366(58)*
Personal	1979						
SD 1st		133 (100)	46 (35)	87 (65)	40 (30)	34 (25)	13 (10)
SD 2nd		75 (100)	5 (7)	70 (93)	13 (17)	26 (35)	31 (41)

*Percentage distribution calculated on 627 total cases in which the number of vessels with critical stenosis where reported.

31%, 11 with thrombus (Baba et al, 1975); 10%, all with thrombus (Warnes et al, 1984) and 4% (Arbustini et al, 1991). In one study (Davies et al, 1984) "plaque fissuring" was present in 103 of 115 vessels showing either mural or occlusive thrombi.

Table 32. Acute occlusive coronary thrombosis in sudden coronary death. Reports in the literature.

Source	Year	Total cases (%)	Thrombus occlusive (%)	Acute infarct (%)	AI + occl. thrombus
Nathanson	1936	142	39 (27)	30 (21)	–
Lisa	1939	41	10 (24)	30 (73)	–
Moritz	1946	115	31 (27)	15 (13)	–
Munck	1946	396	141 (36)	74 (19)	26 (35)
Rabson	1948	617	165 (27)	31 (5)	–
Spain	1959	410	102 (25)	–	–
Branwood	1956	39	14 (36)	–	–
Adelson	1961	500	164 (33)	63 (13)	43 (68)
Crawford	1961	75	39 (52)	24 (32)	–
Franco	1962	187	21 (11)	45 (24)	–
Jorgensen	1968	24	9 (38)	2 (8)	–
Friedman	1973	25 I	1 (4)	0 (0)	–
		34 S	28 (82)	7 (21)	–
Titus	1970	86	13 (15)	34 (39)	–
Spain	1970	189	79 (42)	–	–
Roberts	1972	24	2 (8)	–	–
Scott	1972	183	84 (46)	118 (64)	55 (47)
Liberthson	1975	220	70 (32)	59 (27)	–
Lie	1975	406	69 (17)	148 (36)	–
Kuller	1975	118	30 (25)	13 (11)	–
Baba	1975	121	64 (53)	50 (41)	11 (22)
Reichenbach	1977	87	9 (10)	22 (15)	–
Newman	1982	65	21 (32)	6 (9)	–
Warnes	1984	70	11 (16)	0 (0)	–
Davies	1984	100	44 (44)	– –	
Kragel	1991	21	6 (29)	– –	
Arbustini	1991	27	7 (26)	– –	
Lie	1991	202	36 (18)	63 (31)	–
Total		4524	1309 (29)	834 (22)	*
Personal	1979				
SD 1st		133	11 (8.)	16 (12)	8 (50)
SD 2nd		75	21 (28)	19 (25)	3 (16)

I, instantaneous sudden death; S, sudden death within 24 hours; AI, Acute infarct
* Percentage calculated on the total of 3714 cases in which the frequency of an acute infarct has been reported.

ACUTE MYOCARDIAL NECROSIS

The frequency of acute myocardial infarct necrosis was referred to in 21 studies (Table 32). Infarct size was not considered, but in 7 studies the age of the infarct was estimated histologically (Bedford, 1933; Levy, 1936; Jorgensen et al, 1968; Scott et al, 1972; Liberthson et al, 1975; Baba et al, 1975; Haerem, 1975; Reichenbach et al, 1977). Of these 294 infarcts, 41% were estimated as older than 24 hours. The frequency of an acute occlusive thrombus associated with an infarct ranged from 22-68% (mean 43%) in studies where this variable was reported (Table 32). The frequency of other forms of myocardial necrosis that we define (see chapter 3) was rarely mentioned.

TYPE OF CORONARY DISTRIBUTION

Preponderance of one coronary artery has been considered a pathogenic factor in ischemic heart disease (Schlesinger, 1940). In some studies of sudden coronary death the predominant artery was documented. However, no relation between the type of coronary distribution and sudden death was specified. In general, the left anterior descending branch was the artery more often involved by atherosclerosis and thrombosis in cases of sudden death ("artery of occlusion and sudden death" Barnes et al, 1932), a fact confirmed recently by angiography in patients with ischemic heart disease who subsequently died suddenly (Vlay et al, 1993).

COLLATERALS

Not many systemic postmortem studies on human coronary artery collaterals have been published in the past 25 years. Rather, their presence and distribution has been investigated in patients mainly by cineangiography. This will be discussed in chapter 3. Here it is important to stress that only one previous pathological study investigated intercoronary collaterals in sudden and unexpected death cases (Spain et al, 1963). That study, by postmortem intracoronary injection of calibrated (40 to 75 µm) plastic beads followed by injection of a warmed suspension of barium in gelatin and subsequent histologic examination of the myocardium, indicated the presence of intercoronary collaterals diagnosed by movement of plastic beads from one coronary artery to another; increased X ray vascularity and histologic evidence of giant capillary-like vessels in 10 of 13 SD cases with healed myocardial infarcts and in only 1 of 16 SD cases with advanced coronary atherosclerosis but without infarct. No anastomotic channels were seen in 76 normal subjects with different degrees of coronary atherosclerosis who died by accident. The authors' conclusion was that the absence of collaterals larger than 40 mm might explain sudden death following an acute ischemic attack. The presence of an infarct was believed "a prerequisite for the development of functionally significant intercoronary anastomoses" (Spain et al, 1963).

HEART WEIGHT

In 10 studies (Table 33) the frequency of heart weight following our definition of pathological heart weight ($\geq$500 g) could be calculated. It was 46% amongst 1,279 cases. It is interesting to note that amongst 115 young soldiers who died suddenly (Moritz et al, 1946) none had a pathological heart weight. In reviewing data in these 10 studies it was impossible to correlate heart weight and extensive myocardial fibrosis.

MORPHOLOGIC VARIABLES
OF THE ATHEROSCLEROTIC PLAQUE

Qualitative descriptions of atherosclerotic plaques and the frequency of some morphologic variables have been extensively reported in ischemic heart disease. In particular, in "coronary" sudden death intimal hemorrhage alone or associated with plaque rupture and/or thrombus was investigated in relation to its possible pathogenic meaning. From Table 34 it can be seen that its frequency is, in general, low.

A systematic correlation between different physical and morphologic variables in coronary arteries and postmortem findings in the various clinical patterns of ischemic heart disease is lacking in the literature. Only recently has it been shown that in acute infarction, sudden death and unstable angina patients the mean percent of dense fibrous tissue, calcific deposits and pultaceous debris increases with increasing de-

Table 33. Frequency of pathological heart weight in sudden coronary death. Reports in the literature.

Source	Year	Total cases	Heart Weight 500 g	
			<	$\geq$
Levy	1936	24	4	20
Nathanson	1936	139	104	35
Moritz	1946	115 *	115	0
Adelson	1961	500	170	330
Crawford	1961	75	65	10
Titus	1970	86	41	45
Scott	1972	183	93	90
Kuller	1975	118	76	42
Haerem	1975	33	15	18
Frink	1978	6	6	0
Total		1279 (100%)	689 (54)	590 (46)
Personal	1979			
SD 1st		133	76 (57)	57 (43)
SD 2nd		75	18 (24)	57 (76)

* All soldiers less than 40 yrs old

grees of luminal narrowing while the mean percent of cellular fibrous tissue decreases (Kragel et al, 1989). In other studies active inflammation was significantly related to a reduction of arterial lumen and a cardiac cause of death (Cliff et al, 1988), while a high frequency of T and B lymphocytes was observed in 11 atherosclerotic plaques of patients with unstable angina (100% in the adventitia and 82% in the intima), in 45 plaques of patients with acute myocardial infarction (87% and 91%), in 18 plaques of sudden death cases (72% and 83%) and in 15 plaques of patients dying of noncardiac disease (73% and 65%). In the same study the amount of preserved media, expressed in percentage of the media in histologic sections, was calculated at 10 different levels in each of 90 plaques. The preserved media was 35 ± 9% when a thrombus was present and 29 ± 10% when absent. This difference was not statistically significant (Arbustini et al, 1991).

INTRAMURAL VASCULAR LESIONS

In the literature on sudden coronary death, except for obstructive intimal proliferation of arteries of the conduction system (James, 1985) (see below), functionally significant lesions in the intramural arterial system are limited to platelet aggregates or fibrin-platelet thrombi and/or emboli. A distinction is not made between microthrombi and emboli in small arteries, arterioles, precapillary and capillaries although the latter are related to an acute lesion, e.g., acute thrombus, plaque rupture and acute intimal hemorrhage leading to fibrin-rich emboli in the supplying epicardial artery.

The studies which relate microthrombi or emboli and acute coronary lesions are summarized in Table 35. In all but two of the six (Jorgensen et al, 1968; Haerem et al, 1972) postmortem coronary injection of radiopaque material was performed. A scattered or coalescing myocardial "focal necrosis," defined as "myocytolysis or organized

Table 34. Intimal hemorrhage in sudden coronary death. Reports in the literature.

Source	Year	Total cases	Hemorrhage alone	+ rupt plaque	+ thrombus	+ rupt-th
Jorgensen	1968	24 (100%)	1 (4)	?	?	?
Friedman	1973	25 I	0	0	0	0
		34 S	0	0	0	19 (55)
Liberthson	1974	220	22 (10)	?	?	?
Kuller	1975	169	9 (5)	?	?	?
Baba	1975	121	13 (11)	27 (22)	9 (7)	0
Kragel	1991	21	0	0	0	4 (19)
Arbustini	1991	27	0	0	0	0
Total		641	45 (7)	27 (12)*	9 (4)*	23 (10)*

* Percentage calculated on the total of 228 SD cases in which the various associations were reported.

microinfarcts or myofibrillar lesion" (El-Maraghi et al, 1980); or as "microfocal myocardial necrosis with dark, deeply eosinophilic hypercontracted muscle cells;" or as a "lattice of fine connective stroma at the stage by which necrotic muscle cells have been resorbed" (Davies et al, 1986); or as "recent microinfarcts" consisting of isolated 0.5 mm foci of loose stroma without muscle cells, rich in capillaries, pigment-laden macrophages, lymphocytes and plasma cells (Falk et al, 1985) has been described and linked to intravascular platelet aggregates/thromboemboli. According to Davies et al, (1986) in 23 cases of SD with focal necrosis the latter was associated with platelet aggregates in 65%; in 22 acute infarcts platelet aggregates were found in 75% while in 45 cases without acute myocardial necrosis platelet aggregates were detected in 15%.

In all studies where the conduction system was investigated (Jorgensen et al, 1968; Haerem, 1972; Frink et al, 1978) the frequency of platelet aggregates showed a similar incidence as in other cardiac regions. Atheroemboli with cholesterol crystals were seen in 16 vessels of four cases (Falk, 1985) and in a single vessel in two patients (Davies et al, 1986).

Table 35. Platelet aggregates (PA) fibrin-platelet thrombi (FPT) formed in situ (S) or embolized (E) in sudden coronary death (SD) and "controls" (IHD and/or NC: noncardiac patients). Reports in the literature.

Source	Year	No cases		Survival	Microvasc. lesion (%)	Type	No vessels		subepi ac. lesions	Infarct acute	old	Focal necrosis
Jorgensen	1968	SD	24	<15 m	4 (17)	PAS	"small number"		18	2	0	?
		IHD	78	<48 h	26 (33)				62	44	48	?
Haerem	1971	S D	27	<10 m	23 (85)	PAS	3	(1-22)	10	?	?	?
		IHD	16	months	15 (75)		2	(1-21)	5	?	?	?
		N C	11	?	6 (55)		2	(1-16)	0	0	0	?
Frink	1978	S D	6	?	4 (67)	FPTE	?		6	0	0	?
		N C	3	?	0		?		0	0	0	?
El-Maraghi	1980	S D	50	<24 h	10 (20)	FPTSE	31 ± 31°		8	4	4	10
		IHD	93	>24 h	9 (10)		11 ± 17		7	9	0	0
		Endocar	5	>24 h	5(100)		36 ± 49		0	2	0	6
Falk	1985	S D	25*	<24 h	14 (54)	FPE	72+		25	15 (+ 5?)	0	10
Davies	1986	S D	90	<6 h	27 (30)	PAE	?		26	22** ?		23**
		+ Unstable angina	36		16 (44)		?		?	?	?	?
		No unstable angina	54		11 (20)		?		?	?	?	?

° mainly in subject <45 yr old;

* 26 coronary thrombi in 25 cases;

+ Frequency of microemboli calculated on 26 perfusion territories: 72 in 29 of 260 histo-sections related to thrombosed arteries and 4 emboli in 4 sections not thrombus-related

** 23 with focal necrosis PAE in 15 (65%), 22 with infarct necrosis PAE in 16 (75%), 45 without necrosis PAE in 6 (15%)

CONDUCTION SYSTEM

The complexity of studying the conduction system by serial or semiserial section study limited its examination to a few investigations. One is represented by 30 clinicopathologic papers ("De Subitaneis Mortibus") published in *Circulation* from August 1975 to June 1978 (James et al, 1973-1978; Brechenmacher et al, 1976,1977). Amongst 77 sudden death cases reported, 60 were associated by the authors with different underlying diseases, seven with conduction disturbances (varying degrees of heart block, paroxysmal atrial fibrillation, premature ventricular beats, etc.) and 10 had no history of associated disease or precursor episodes (Table 36). The pathologic findings observed in the 77 cases are presented in Table 37.

Another study (Lie, 1975) examined the conduction system from 35 men and 14 women (mean age 57 and 62 years respectively) with ischemic heart disease. The subjects, 39 with, and 10 without histologically demonstrated myocardial infarcts, died suddenly within 6 hours of their acute symptoms developing. Most hearts had severe (>75% cross sectional area) coronary atherosclerosis and acute ischemia expressed by myofibrillar degeneration and cardiomegaly (>350 g). Forty percent of cases in both groups had a healed myocardial infarction while a recent coronary thrombus was demonstrated in 18% of infarct and 20% of noninfarct cases. Findings in the conduction system of all cases were intimal thickening with severe luminal stenosis of the sinoatrial artery in 26% or of the atrioventricular node artery in 52%; destruction of the atrioventricular node in 2 instances with massive interventricular septal infarction, fibrosis and/or fatty replacement of sinus node (9 cases), atrioventricular node (2), His bundle (22), and

Table 36. Serial section study of the conduction system—Underlying disease in 77 cases reported by TN James et al.

Disease	No Cases
Hypertrophic cardiomyopathy	22
Scleroderma	8
Long QT syndrome	8
Rupture of infarcted IV septum	5
Pheochromocytoma	3
Type A Woff-Parkinson-White syndrome	2
Persisting superior vena cava	2
Rheumathoid arthritis	2
Pickwickian syndrome - Homocystinuria	
Familial congenital heart block - Whipple's disease	
Ankylosing spondilitis -Sarcoidosis	
Coarctation of aorta - Metastatic hypernephroma	1 each
Idiopathic conduction disturbances	7
No history	10

Table 37. Serial section study of the conduction system—Pathological findings in 77 cases reported by TN James et al.

Pathological findings	No cases
1. Benign tumor (fibroma, Purkinje cell, polycystic AV)	4
2. Fibromuscular medial dysplasia sinus/AV node arteries	
no underlying disease	6
hypertrophic cardiomyopathy	13
scleroderma	7
pheochromocytoma	3
IV septum rupture (infarct)	3
homocystinuria - rheumatoid arthritismyocarditis - sarcoidosis - ankylosing spondylitis coarctation of aorta	6 each
3. Anomalies of conduction system (persistent fetal dispersion or malformations AV node/His bundle, unusual connections, venous lacunae, etc.)	25
4. Focal neuritis and neural degeneration (Long QT syndrome)	8
5. Focal or diffuse replacement by adipose tissue	12
6. Focal degeneration or fibrosis	35
7. Panarteritis (Whipple's disease)	1
8. Disseminated intravascular coagulation	1
9. Platelet aggregates (pheochromocytoma, homocystimuria)	4
10. Fibromuscular polypoid mass occluding SN artery	1
11. Severe coronary atherosclerosis	10
12. Atresia left main trunk with diffuse myocarditis	1

of right (4) or left (14) or both bundle branches (7). Dysplasia of the atrioventricular node artery was present in 44% of 27 sudden death cases vs 6% of 17 controls in another study (Burke et al, 1993). Sudden death was associated with exercise in half of these individuals.

Finally in his study, Rossi (1982) included 13 cases who died "suddenly and unexpectedly from the initial symptoms of myocardial infarction." The latter was documented in 9 subjects, one with Buerger's disease and the others with coronary atherosclerosis, while 2 had panarteritis nodosa, 1 aortic insufficiency and 1 apparently had no significant autopsy findings in any organ. Severe (>70%) obstruction ("fibromuscular dysplasia") or occlusive thrombosis of the sinoatrial artery was seen in 1 and 3 cases respectively. In the atrioventricular node artery these figures were 4 and 0 cases. The sinoatrial arterial thrombosis was associated with panarteritis nodosa in 2 cases and Buerger disease in 1. "Ischemic abnormalities" such as myofibrillar degeneration with contraction bands or idiopathic fibrosis, were present in all but 1 case. In particular, an extensive infarct (1 case) or widespread ischemic degeneration and fibrosis in the sinoatrial node (2 cases) and patchy degeneration/necrosis, edema, leukocytic infiltration in the atrioventricular node (1 case), common bundle (1 case) or bundle branches (5 cases) were recorded. Twelve of the 13 hearts revealed neural abnormalities marked by vacuolar swelling of nerve sheaths, epiperineural edema, inflammation, hemorrhage or congestion with disruption of axons and/or neural degeneration, neural interstitial fibrosis, proliferation of ganglionic capsular (satellite) cells with neuronal loss (Terplan or Nageotte nodules). Two stellate ganglia surgically removed in two other patients with myocardial infarction associated with recurrent bursts of ventricular fibrillation showed similar changes. Degeneration of neural element in sudden death has been reported by James, (1986); Rossi, (1985) and Shvalev, (1986).

SUDDEN CORONARY DEATH AND EXERCISE

The risk of strenuous exercise in ischemic heart disease is controversial (Gibbons et al, 1987). A review of studies (Table 32) where "physical effort" at the time of sudden death was investigated (2,324 cases) shows that death occurs mainly while a patient is at rest or sleeping or during minimal activity (69%). The remaining 707 subjects were at work.

In this, pathologic findings observed in selected groups such as young athletes and joggers who die suddenly must be mentioned. Amongst 78 athletes reported (Heath, 1969; Opie, 1975; Noakes et al, 1979a, 1979b; Maron et al, 1980; Morales et al, 1980; Waller et al, 1980; Tsung et al, 1982; Virmani et al, 1982b; Voigt et al, 1982; Thiene et al, 1983, 1985) the pathology found at autopsy was mainly cardiac (Table 38) and generally related to chronic disease. Only in 3 cases, 1 with pulmonary thromboembolism and two with rupture of the aorta was an acute event possibly linked with the death. The age distribution of these 78 cases (Table 39) shows that coronary atherosclerosis was estimated a cause of death in 3% under the age of 20 years, in 40% between 20-29, in 67% between 30-39 and 100% after 40 years. Similarly in 36 joggers (Morales et al, 1980; Virmani et al, 1982b; Thiene et al, 1985) who died suddenly (Table 40) coronary atherosclerosis was the estimated cause of sudden death in 92%.

Some of these cases seem appropriate to discuss regarding the functional significance of pathologic findings (see chapter 4). For instance, that of a 12-year-old girl (Heath, 1969) who suddenly died following a swimming race, without any history of cardiac symptoms or signs despite her active athletic life; or the two following cases of marathon runners (Noakes et al, 1979a):

1. A 44-year-old male, nonsmoker, who had been running for 14 months completed 8 standard 42 km marathons, a 56 km race in 5 hours and 59 minutes and a 90 km marathon in 10 hours and 10 minutes. In training he ran 48 to 80 km per week. He had no history of ischemic heart disease. Following a 50-km race (4 hours and 59 minutes) and, 1 month later, a standard 42-km marathon (4 hours and 2 minutes) he visited a general practitioner complaining of a

"nonspecific lack of energy." There were no symptoms or signs of ischemic heart disease and all tests were negative. No electrocardiogram was performed. Shortly afterward he competed in a 24-km race. At the 19-km mark, while running without distress, he stopped to adjust a loose shoelace. Bending down, he suddenly lost consciousness and died instantaneously.

At autopsy the main findings were: heart weight 357 g; extensive old antero-septal scar (old "silent" infarct); grade 4 (75-100%) lumen reduction in the first 5 mm of the left coronary descending branch and associated total oc-

Table 38. Pathology in 78 athletes who died suddenly. Reports in the literature.

Pathology	M	W	Tot.	Age	Heart Weight	History	Physical activity	Other
Anomalous origin cor. artery	7	–	7	17-22 19	450-480 465	no	6	1 + hypertr. cardiomyopathy
Hypoplasia right cor. artery	–	1	1	17	280	no	no	–
"Mural" left ant. descending branch	–	1	1	17	260	no	1	Reflow necrosis coag. myocyt.
Hypertrophic cardiomyopathy	13	2	15	13-30 18	360-650 561	7	?	Thickening septal arteries
Floppy mitral valve	3	–	3	17-27 22	420-530 475	2	2	1+fibromusc.hyper – AV node artery
Idiopathic LV hypertrophy	4	–	4	16-28 19	420-465 448	no	4	1+fibromusc.hyper – AV node artery
Heart tumor	1	1	2	12-15 14	?	1	2	one fibroma one myxoma
Ruptured aorta	2	–	2	18-21 19	?	2	2	Medial cystic necrosis
Lung thrombo-embolism	–	1	1	20	?	no	?	–
Anomaly conduct. system	1	1	2	11-35 23	?	no	?	–
Right ventr. dysplasia	7	–	7	16-26 21	410-540 502	4	7	–
Atherosclerosis coronary	33	–	33	17-58 38	345-480 406	16	14	–

References quoted in the text

clusion by organized and recanalized thrombus. The other severe (75-100%) coronary lesion found was 3.5 cm from the origin of the left circumflex branch. There was no evidence of a fresh infarction but foci of "contraction band necrosis" were present in both ventricles. The conduction system was normal.

2. A 41-year-old man who had been a marathon runner for 2 years, suffered an acute myocardial infarction. He had a complete angiographic occlusion of the left circumflex branch, 50% narrowing of the proximal tract of the right coronary artery and minor luminal irregularities of the left descending vessel (March 1976). Ignoring medical advice and after appropriate training, approximately 1 year after his infarction, he completed a 50-km race in 5 hours and 36 minutes. Two weeks later he ran a 42-km marathon in 4 hours 45 minutes, followed by 3 additional marathons in

Table 39. Cardiovascular pathology related to their age in 78 athletes who died suddenly. Reports in the literature.

Pathology	<20	20-29	30-39	>40	Total
Anomalous origin cor. arteries	5 (17%)	2 (8%)	–	–	7 (9%)
Hypoplasia right cor. artery	1 (3)	–	–	–	1 (1)
"Mural" left ant. desc. branch	1 (3)	–	–	–	1 (1)
Hypertrophic cardiomyopathy	10 (34)	4 (16)	1 (17)	–	15 (19)
Floppy mitral valve	1 (3)	2 (8)	–	–	3 (4)
Idiopathic LV hypertrophy	3 (10)	1 (4)	–	–	4 (5)
Heart tumor	2 (7)	–	–	–	2 (3)
Ruptured aorta	1 (3)	1 (4)	–	–	2 (3)
Lung thrombo-embolism	–	1 (4)	–	–	1 (1)
Anomaly conduct. system	1 (3)	–	1 (17)	–	2 (3)
Right ventr. dysplasia	3 (10)	4 (16)	–	–	7 (9)
Coronary atherosclerosis	1 (3)	10 (40)	4 (66)	18 (100)	33 (42)
Total	29 (100)	25 (100)	6 (100)	18 (100)	78 (100)

References quoted in the text

Table 40. Pathology in 36 joggers who died suddenly. Reports in the literature.

Pathology	M	W	Tot.	Age (yrs)	Heart Weight (g)	History	Physical activity
G.I. hemorrhage	1	–	1	28	?	no	?
"Mural" coronary artery	2	–	2	34-54	400-460	1	2
Coronary atherosclerosis	33	–	33	18-58	?	13	33

References quoted in the text

the following 3 months. From the time of infarction to his last race (28 months) he ran 3,624 km. Pain in the chest, jaw or left arm occurred several times during training runs but he did not seek medical advice. Subsequently, he was readmitted to hospital for 2 episodes of unstable angina. Angiography confirmed the complete occlusion of the left circumflex and revealed total occlusion of the right coronary artery and 80% stenosis of the left anterior descending branch (October 1978). While awaiting coronary bypass surgery, he began to have severe chest pain. Electrocardiography suggested an acute myocardial infarction with acute anterolateral ST-segment elevation and increasing size of Q waves in V_5 and V_6. Despite therapy the heart stopped within 30 minutes and resuscitation failed. There was no evidence of serum enzyme changes.

At autopsy the heart (349 g) showed: grade 4 (75-100%) obstruction in the first tracts of the left anterior descending, left circumflex branches and the right coronary artery, with superimposed fresh thrombus in the left descending, organized thrombus of the left circumflex and organizing thrombus of the right coronary artery. A healed infarct of the left ventricular inferior wall, its appearance in keeping with one suffered 2 years before, was documented. An acute myocardial infarction was not demonstrated but foci of contraction band necrosis were observed. The conduction system was normal.

Finally three sudden death cases with a "mural" left anterior descending branch and strenuous exercise (Morales et al, 1980) deserve attention (Noble et al, 1976):

1. For many years a 54-year-old man had episodic left precordial pain radiating to his back, emotional stress especially induced it. ECG demonstrated subendocardial ischemia with a strongly positive exercise stress test. Coronary angiogram showed a "milking effect" in the proximal portion of the left anterior descending vessel. Ventricular function was normal. He died suddenly while jogging.

   Pathological findings were limited to the heart. It weighed 440 g. A 2.5 x 1.3 cm scar with intermixed brown myocardium involved the most anterior portion of the ventricular septum and adjacent left anterior ventricular wall from the apex to within 2.5 cm of the base. Coronary arteries showed only two plaques with 50% lumen reduction of the posterior right coronary artery and first segment of the left descending branch. Two centimeters from its origin the left circumflex was covered (for 4.5 cm) by a loop of atrial muscle while the left anterior descending immediately after the atherosclerotic plaque dipped into the myocardium for 3 cm. Histologically, patchy irregular areas of healing necrosis alternated with areas of normal or injured ("muscle with irregular outlines, myocytolysis, fragmentation") myocardium in the anterior septum and left ventricular wall. The atrioventricular nodal branch was stenosed by concentric intimal hyperplasia.

2. A 34-year-old man without a medical history died suddenly while jogging. The heart weighed 460 g. Three and a half centimeters from its origin the left anterior descending coronary branch showed a "mural" disposition for 2 cm. No atherosclerosis was found in coronary arteries. Grossly and histologically myocardial changes were similar to that described in case 1.

3. A 17-year-old women was swimming in a pool. After completing approximately 10 laps, she helped herself from the pool but immediately thereafter became unconscious, with no vital signs. She died in hospital 14 hours after resuscitation attempts. Autopsy findings were marked congestion and edema of the lungs. The heart (260 g) was free of coronary lesions. The right coronary artery was overbridged for 3 cm in its posterior tract. At its origin the left anterior descending branch dipped into the myocardium for 2 cm and for 1.5 cm in its terminal segment. The endocardial half of the entire left ventricle was dark red with a histological pattern of hemorrhagic necrosis where necrotic myocardial fibers, often with contraction bands, were spread apart by interstitial hemorrhage and an early polymorphonuclear leucocytic infiltrate. No myocardial fibrosis was present.

Faruqui et al, (1978) reported the successful surgical treatment of patients with ischemic heart disease by debridging.

CHAPTER 3

NATURAL HISTORY OF ISCHEMIC HEART DISEASE

History provides knowledge of events and their relationships and may allow interpretation of many subsequent phenomena. So too in science, knowledge is built upon a steady, historical accumulation of facts. In medicine such knowledge is a prerequisite to rationally prevent and treat diseases. It implies first, that all variables which have a role in the clinical history are recognized and second, that correct explanations of their cause/effect relationships are available in the different phases of a disease including prodromata, onset, clinical course, recovery or death.

For a pathologist the tools of reconstructing or discovering a disease's natural history are pathologic signs observed at autopsy and, to a lesser extent, in biopsy material. Unfortunately, the latter often offer a limited spatial and chronological view while the former present end results with the very difficult, sometimes impossible, task of understanding pathophysiologic evolution and the cause of death. On the other hand, only the pathologist can outline structural changes to explain dysfunction and may follow the natural history of any morphologic sign in the general population. In part, these limits of human pathology may be surpassed by experimental pathology, more and more linked with biochemistry and molecular biology. However, the results of experimental studies must always be interpreted in light of observed morphologic or pathophysiologic changes in human beings. Imaging, too, has been added to our armamentarium to help understand disease, but its application in vivo is usually confined to a population selected by disease. Despite a present tendency to underestimate the value of pathology, we need all of these approaches to study disease. Structure and function form a unit and the old dictum *"Mors gaudet succurrere vitae"* (death helps life), is still valid; particularly to understand the meaning of any symptom or sign in the history of a disease.

In chapter 3 we review the natural history of some morphologic patterns, which, at present, are of paramount importance in attempting to define *ischemic* heart disease in general and sudden *coronary* death in particular.

NATURAL HISTORY OF THE ATHEROSCLEROTIC PLAQUE—BLOOD VESSELS AND HEMODYNAMICS

Blood vessels are sensitive structures which respond to hemodynamic changes. Thus, endothelial nuclear shape and orientation, e.g., elongated, flow-direction oriented nuclei in segments with stable flow round, less ordered nuclei in segments with unsteady, turbulent flow, and possibly the density of endothelial nuclei depend upon stresses secondary to flow dynamics (Flaherty et al, 1972). In general, the architecture of a vessel wall is proportionate to the latter (Burton, 1954) and may change according to the nature of variations in flow dynamics (Rodbard, 1971). Types of stresses which act on the vessel wall are *compressional* with a radial direction; *tensile* with circumferential and longitudinal directions and *shearing* which depends on flow velocity and viscosity and is caused by the drag of flowing blood acting parallel to the vascular surface (Fry, 1969). When stresses reach a critical point, structural changes can be expected in the vessel wall (Langille, 1991). In particular, an increase in shear stress stimulates vasodilation in normal coronary arteries, limiting this stress at the endothelial surface. This is in contrast to atherosclerotic arteries in which vasodilation is reduced and major shear stress can be expected (Vita et al, 1989).

Human coronary arteries may be divided into two functionally divergent systems in relation to cardiac and flow dynamics, the extra- and intramural vessels. They appear to be good models in which to study the relationship of flow dynamics and atherogenesis. In extramural arteries a distinction must be drawn between (a) *physiological intimal thickening;* (b) *nonatherosclerotic obliterative intimal thickening* and (c) *segmental atherosclerotic obstructive intimal thickening* based on clear-cut structural aspects induced by each of these types of intimal processes.

PHYSIOLOGICAL AND PATHOLOGICAL CHANGES IN HUMAN EXTRAMURAL CORONARY ARTERIES

PHYSIOLOGICAL INTIMAL THICKENING

Normally, the intima of extramural coronary arteries shows a histologic pattern not seen, or at least not as well developed, in other muscular arteries (Fig. 2). Although the role of this change in the pathogenesis of atherosclerosis is controversial, the finding must be distinguished from changes seen in atherosclerotic plaques (Silver et al, 1980; Angelini et al, 1990; Baroldi, 1991a). It consists of an intimal thickening starting at birth (Bork, 1926; Dock, 1946) and undergoing progressive changes with age. According to Wolkoff (1929), two

layers more or less divided by an elastic lamina are readily recognizable in the first decade of life. The outer one, defined as *elastic-mus-
cular* is formed by the splitting of the internal elastic membrane and
by a proliferation of medial smooth muscle fibers through fenestra-
tions in the latter. These proliferating smooth muscle fibers assume a
generally longitudinal disposition. The inner or *elastic hyperplastic* layer
is formed by elastic fibers derived from the separating lamina. It must
be noted that in the first decade of life, such intimal thickening frequently does not exceed the width of the media. It is more prominent
at branching sites, does not generally involve the whole vessel circumference and shows a great variability in different subjects and in different segments of the same vessel, being more prominent in men than
women (Dock, 1946; Fangman et al, 1947; Moon, 1957; Schornagel,
1956). In particular, Dock (1946) found a three-fold greater frequency
of this intimal thickening in male newborns, a finding not confirmed
by Minkowski, (1947) who was able to observe a greater frequency in
males only in subjects older than one month or in subsequent decades
of life. A thickening of the *elastic hyperplastic* layer occurs with the
appearance of a subendothelial fibrous layer which becomes prominent after the fourth decade. Intimal thickening at this time may exceed medial thickness (Wolkoff, 1929; French et al, 1962; Geer et al,
1968; Likar et al, 1969; Vlodaver et al, 1967a, 1968a).

As in the evolution of myocardial hypertrophy (Meerson, 1969),
it is possible to recognize three stages in the evolution of this physiological intimal thickening caused by hemodynamic stresses: (1) *an
early change* characterized by proliferation in the intima of medial
myocytes and elastic lamellar splitting; (2) *a stable, hyperfunctioning
stage,* mainly characterized by myocellular hyperplasia from the media
and a fibroelastic hyperplasia; (3) *an exhaustion stage,* in which the
intima becomes fibrotic. In this proliferative response, the predominant role of medial smooth muscle cells has been interpreted as that
of a *multifunctional medial mesenchymal cell* capable of contraction,
proliferation, migration, colonization and synthesis of collagen, elas-
tin, ground substance and basement membrane material (Wissler, 1967).

Physiological intimal thickening has been interpreted by some as
early atherosclerotic damage (Ehrich et al, 1931; Fangman et al, 1947;
Moon, 1957) or, alternatively as being secondary to (1) an inflamma-
tory/allergic processes (Minkowski, 1947); (2) platelet microthrombi
deposition (Likar et al, 1969), or (3) to hemodynamic stress (Spalteholz
et al, 1931; Schornagel, 1956; Vlodaver et al, 1967a; Baroldi, 1969).
Such circumferential intimal thickening, normally found in adults, can
be considered a component of postnatal vasogenesis (Vlodaver al, 1967a)
related to the peculiar flow dynamics in extramural coronary arteries,
i.e., systolic filling without or with minor intramural discharge due to
myocardial systolic contraction; which increases all types of wall stress.
It is not necessarily associated with true atherosclerotic change. Variations

in the degree of intimal thickening in different subjects most likely depend upon individual variations in flow dynamics. Their importance is confirmed by the absence of such intimal thickening in the intramural arterial system and in those tracts of extramural coronary arteries covered by myocardial bridges ("Mural coronary artery" after Geiringer, 1951a) (Fig. 3). We presume that systolic contraction of the latter counteracts the action of dynamic stresses on the arterial wall resulting in no tridimensional expansion and annulling proliferative response. However, we cannot exclude that a different intensity of neural, possibly adrenergic, control on arterial wall tone may play a determining role. This may explain divergencies amongst individuals, different ethnic groups (Vlodaver et al, 1969) and species with a similar distribution of extramural coronary arteries. For example, we have not seen in dogs the physiologic coronary intimal thickening reported in humans or other animals (French et al, 1962; Geer et al, 1968).

NONATHEROSCLEROTIC OBLITERATIVE INTIMAL THICKENING

Nonatherosclerotic obliterative intimal thickening is a diffuse pathologic process of unknown nature which affects the whole intima of extramural coronary arteries. It may produce extremely severe concentric stenosis of vessels and is observed in conditions, such as (a) coarctation of the aorta (Vlodaver et al, 1968b); (b) transplanted human hearts (Thomson, 1969; Cooley et al, 1969; Bieber et al, 1970; Smith et al, 1987; Billingham, 1988; Baroldi, 1991a, Rose et al, 1991); (c) transplanted dog hearts (Kosek et al, 1969) (Fig. 4) and (d) in aortocoronary saphenous vein grafts (Johnson et al, 1970; Marti et al, 1971; Vlodaver et al, 1971; Brody et al, 1972; Kern et al, 1972; Virmani et al, 1991) (Fig. 5). We note that similar intimal/medial changes have also been observed in vessels of other organs in a variety of both human and experimental conditions such as hypertension (Spiro et al, 1965; Oka et al, 1967; Esterly et al, 1968; Cohn et al, 1970; Still, 1968; Constantinides, 1970; Huttner et al, 1970; Wolinski, 1972), following catecholamine administration (Szakacs et al, 1959), by varying flow volume (Rodbard, 1956; Hassler, 1970; Schaper et al, 1972), as a result of trauma (Hassler, 1970) and in specific degenerative, e.g., juvenile intimal sclerosis, or infectious/immune diseases, e.g., rheumatic fever.

This obliterative intimal thickening has been interpreted as a variant of atherosclerosis. Some investigators, wrongly in our opinion (see below), speak of "accelerated atherosclerosis" affecting vein grafts (Bulkley et al, 1977) and coronary arteries in transplanted hearts. Long-term survivors of cardiac transplantation (Graham et al, 1972; Rider et al, 1972), as well as experimental cardiac allografts where animals are fed a cholesterol rich diet (Alonzo et al, 1970), develop atheromatous deposits in this intimal thickening. However, the latter is likely a late, secondary process that has been linked to toxic antibodies and hyperlipidemia (Hess et al, 1983), to lymphostasis (Mehmet et al, 1987) or to cyclosporine and prednisone therapy (Uretsky et al, 1987). As dynamic factors appear important in the pathogenesis of atherosclerosis it is not surprising that intimal thickening and atherosclerosis may have a similar location. However, idiopathic obliterative intimal thickening, even in its last subocclusive stage is a result of proliferation of smooth muscle cells with minimal or absent elastic hyperplasia, increased ground substance (proteoglycans) and interstitial fibrosis. The internal elastic membrane is intact and not one of the morphologic variables, i.e., hemorrhage, vascularization, atheroma, calcification, lympho-plasmacellular inflammation of the atherosclerotic plaque is obvious, except in late stages.

"Acceleration" of a process means that its history occurs in a shorter period than usual. However, all components of the process must be present. If not, the process is a distinct entity with its own history. One notes that nonatherosclerotic obliterative intimal thickening often occurs in denervated vessels as in transplanted hearts or vein grafts suggesting a possible role for the loss of the neurogenic control on vessel wall tone. In relating this change to an effect of cyclosporine one should recall that the obliterative intimal process was observed in the precyclosporine era of heart transplantation (Thomson, 1969; Cooley et al, 1969). Both physiologic and idiopathic obliterative intimal thickening, particularly in subjects at risk, may predispose a vessel to atherosclerosis.

ATHEROSCLEROTIC INTIMAL THICKENING

Atherosclerotic intimal thickening (Fig. 6) is mainly a segmental lesion with complications that involve the media and adventitia (Strong et al, 1968). Our findings seem to indicate that coronary atherosclerosis evolves mainly in adult age with minimal or no further progression in the elderly (Table 5). In chapter 1 the morphologic variables of this process in ischemic cardiac patients and in the normal general population were described. We constructed a history of the coronary atherosclerotic plaque by studying many coronary sections and verifying the trend of morphological changes in relation to intimal thickening and lumen reduction in ischemic and clinically normal subjects. From the significant associations of first and second order of variables and the highest chi-square values obtained according to sensitive and specific codes (see section on statistical methods), it was possible to outline a tridimensional, i.e., radial, circumferential, longitudinal progression of the atherosclerotic plaque in patients with ischemic heart disease and in controls (Table 41). It is as follows: initially a plaque is a nodular fibrous intimal thickening likely due to smooth muscle cell hyperplasia with subsequent fibrous tissue replacement. This early fibrous plaque is the only pattern occasionally seen in young people less than 20 years old (Angelini et al, 1990). The second stage is proteoglycan accumulation (basophilia) deep to the fibrous cap. Both fibrosis and basophilia are recurrent phenomena being two basic elements in plaque progression. Subsequently, foam cells and cholesterol clefts and/or calcification appear in the proteoglycan pool, in keeping with the chemical affinity of glycosaminoglycans for lipoproteins and calcium salts (Wight et al, 1983). Therefore, a basophilic pool may evolve either into a calcified area or atheroma. The final plaque pattern is a result of the extension in three directions of these repetitive phenomena (Fig. 7A,B) plus further complications including hemorrhage, thrombosis, etc. (Fig. 7C-E). It is a pattern (Morgan, 1956; McGill et al, 1968; Velican et al, 1989) different to that seen in the experimental plaque resulting from a diet rich in cholesterol, or in familial hypercholesterolemia (Fig. 7F).

Nevertheless, several points in this history are still obscure. For example, the factor(s) which promote smooth cell hyperplasia (platelet growth factors, Ross, 1979; catecholamines, etc., Velican et al, 1989) the nature of cells participating in plaque growth, whether endothelial, smooth muscle, monocyte/macrophages, histiocytes or a unique mesenchymal multifunctional cell capable of transforming structure and endocrine activity according to functional need and the role of hemodynamic stresses all need further clarification. An impressive example of the importance of hemodynamic stresses is provided by adult patients with an anomalous origin of one coronary artery from the pulmonary artery with its low flow pressure and pulsation. In this condition, the anomalous artery is free of atherosclerosis whereas the other, arising from the aorta, may be severely atherosclerotic (Kaunitz, 1947;

Table 41. Progression of atherosclerotic plaque in relation to increasing intimal thickness and lumen reduction

Intimal thickness μ	Morphologic variables	Lumen reduction %
> 300	Nodular smooth myocellular hyperplasia ↓ fibrosis	< 50
600	Fibrosis + basophilia early advential/intimal inflammatory reaction	50-69
1000 ↓ ≥ 2000	Basophilia Atheroma ↑ Calcification ↑ Inflammatory reaction	70-79 ↓ > 90

Burch et al, 1962; Blake et al, 1964). These patients have unique genetic and environmental backgrounds. The only difference to explain findings are different flow dynamics in the two coronary arteries. Again, diphasic flow dynamics may stimulate the neural control of the vessel wall responsible for its morphologic changes. Unanswered questions relate to the variability in location of atherosclerotic plaques in the coronary system, despite some preferential sites of formation. In other words, how do etiologic factors act preferentially in vascular segments of one subject while in others different segments are involved, despite an apparently similar wall structure and hemodynamics?

The effects of intimal vascularization on plaque formation are also unknown. In our study, which was in partial agreement with that of Geiringer, (1951b), vascularization was present in 24% of sections with an intimal thickness between 300 and 599 μm. Its frequency was maximal (75%) with a thickness between 600 and 1,999 μm, and was a little less with greater intimal thickness. However vascularization was mild in the majority of sections (61%). Our data suggest that it follows plaque formation and cannot be interpreted (Barger et al, 1984) as an important factor in plaque growth. Furthermore, in our experience, the possibility that neovascularization is the result of the organization of mural thrombi (Morgan, 1956) can be considered only when found in severe stenoses (for serial section findings see below).

INFLAMMATION

Another variable of the atherosclerotic plaque is the inflammatory reaction. Its role in atherogenesis must be clarified. A current theory, arising from study of the experimental plaque in hypercholesterolemic animals, states that atherosclerosis: "results from an excessive inflammatory—fibroproliferative response to various forms of insult to the endothelium and smooth muscle of (the) artery wall. ...The earliest recognizable lesion is the so called 'fatty streak', an aggregation of lipid-muscle macrophages and T lymphocytes within the inner most layer of the artery wall, the intima... (The) macrophage is the principal inflammatory mediator of cells, acting not only as an antigen-presenting cells to T lymphocytes but also a scavenger cell to remove noxious materials and as (a) source of growth regulatory molecules and cytokines." (Ross, 1993) In contrast are the lymphocytic and plasma cell infiltrates we observed in human plaques from the general population and ischemic patients. They appear to be a distinct inflammatory response to a still unknown agent (Fig. 6G). Long described in the literature (Morgan, 1956; Kochi et al, 1985; Velican et al, 1989) they were considered a minor complication related to plaque size (Schwartz et al, 1962) and possibly to reduction of arterial lumen, or interpreted as to an autoimmune process (plasma cell cytoplasm stained with IgG and IgM antisera; Parums et al, 1981; Wal et al, 1989). In our experience this inflammatory infiltrate forms during "proteoglycan accumulation" stage of the plaque, being visible in 32% and 62% respectively of mild

(<50%) and moderate (50-69%) luminal stenoses and with an intimal thickening between 300-599 µm. The "historical" importance of this lesion is its significantly higher frequency, extension and strategic location around advential nerves adjacent to the media, in patients with ischemic heart disease than in healthy people with an equal degree of coronary stenosis and intimal thickening. Finally, the prevalence of short (≤3 mm) severe stenoses in AMI patients may indicate that this inflammation, always found in these subjects, may influence the radial progression of a plaque (Baroldi, 1985a, Baroldi et al, 1988; Cliff et al, 1988).

INTIMAL HEMORRHAGE

Intimal hemorrhage is a real event in the natural history of a coronary atherosclerotic plaque (Fig. 6F) and has been considered the possible source of lipoprotein material, vasoactive substance and thrombogenic factors (Patterson, 1938; Morgan, 1956; Velican et al, 1989) or to cause occlusion (Wartman, 1938). Intimal vascularization is a potential source of intimal hemorrhage although Davies et al, (1984) provided this contrary opinion: "... we have avoided the term 'plaque hemorrhage' since it is a source of confusion. 'Plaque fissuring' is the term applied to the formation of an opening from the lumen into the intima; it leads to what was known originally as 'dissecting hemorrhage' but is actually an intraintimal thrombus not just red cells but mainly fibrin and platelets."

Intimal hemorrhage was observed in 21% of cases with unstable angina, 19% of sudden death and 63% of acute infarct cases in one study (Kragel et al, 1991). In ours it was the variable with the lowest total frequency (14%) and with the lowest frequency at any level of lumen reduction or intimal thickness. In 289 sections with intimal hemorrhage, 48% were in the infarct-related artery.

PLAQUE RUPTURE

Plaque rupture (Fig. 7C) is another parameter to be considered in natural history. It affects atheromatous "rupture-prone" plaques and is generated by tiny fissures at the periphery of the fibrous cap that covers the plaque's lipid-rich core (Falk, 1992). At this location the plaque is thinner and infiltrated by macrophages. Intimal macrophage inflammation has been proposed as a possible mechanism of plaque fissuring (Buja et al, 1994; Moreno et al, 1994; Wal et al, 1989, 1994). Plaque rupture may result in occlusion of the lumen by releasing pultaceous material, already reported by Branwood (1956) or be associated with overlying thrombus formation (Osborn, 1963; Friedman et al, 1966; Constantinides, 1970; Ridolfi et al, 1977). In our study we did not serially section all examined plaques. Therefore, we have no exact figures about the frequency of plaque rupture. However, coronary occlusion by pultaceous material alone was an exceptional finding and always associated with hemorrhage or thrombus at a different plaque level. A thrombus with subintimal expansion through a break in the intima was also a rare finding.

Plaque fissuring was reported in 89% of 115 coronary vessels with an associated mural or occlusive thrombus in one study (Davies et al, 1984) and in 81% of 25 vessels in another (Falk, 1985). In other studies plaque rupture per se was observed in 36% of cases with unstable angina, 19% with sudden death and 75% with acute myocardial infarct (Kragel et al, 1991); or was absent in cases with unstable and stable angina and present in 7% of cases with acute myocardial infarction, 4% with sudden death, 12% with congestive heart failure and 7% of control cases (Arbustini et al, 1991). Keep in mind that by coronary angioscopy 60-80% of patients with unstable angina have complicated atheromata, i.e., rupture, ulceration, thrombus formation (Sherman et al, 1986; Forrester et al, 1987; Hombach et al, 1988).

MEDIAL CHANGES

The type, frequency and extension of tunica media damage at the site of an atherosclerotic plaque are all important factors in relation to coronary artery spasm; a point that has been poorly investigated. In our experience, medial changes were seen only at the plaque site and are marked by thickness reduction in concentric plaques. Occasionally, focal destruction associated with inflammatory reaction was observed. In another study a reduction of 70% of the medial area was calculated at plaque level (Arbustini et al, 1991).

PLAQUE REGRESSION

A concept pertinent to the natural history of the atherosclerotic plaque is its regression. This has not been studied specifically in our investigations. A reduction or disappearance of luminal stenosis has been reported occasionally in coronary angiographic studies (Bemis et al, 1973; Gensini et al, 1972; Laks et al, 1979; Rafflenbeul et al, 1979; Haft et al, 1993) and interpreted as recanalization of a thrombus, lysis of an embolus (O' Reilly et al, 1974) or resolution of vasoconstriction or spasm. However, regression of angiographic lesions and reduction of clinical events, i.e., death, infarction, worsening symptoms, were obtained by intensive lipid-lowering therapy in patients with high levels of apolipoprotein B, documented ischemic heart disease and a family history of vascular disease (Brown et al, 1990). Furthermore, the reduction of an experimental lesion after suspension of an atherogenic diet (Wissler, 1978) and the practical absence of advanced atherosclerotic plaques in cachectic people raises the possibility of plaque regression (see below where different types of atherosclerotic plaque are discussed).

In the International Nifedipine Trial on Antiatherosclerotic Therapy, regression marked by a decrease in percent diameter of stenoses ≥20% was observed in only 4% of 1,063 coronary segments when 348 patients with moderately advanced coronary atherosclerosis, i.e., one or few coronary stenoses or occlusion in only one major vessel were studied by quantitative coronary angiography performed 3 years apart (Jost et al, 1993). In this study progression of coronary obstruction occurred in segments greater than 2 mm in diameter in a proximal or midartery position and in the right coronary artery.

NATURAL HISTORY OF CORONARY OCCLUSION IN ISCHEMIC HEART DISEASE

At present three forms of subepicardial coronary occlusion are described in ischemic heart disease. One is functional, due to contraction of the tunica media (*spasm*) and the other two morphological with occlusion of the lumen by either a thrombus or by pultaceous material following rupture of an atheroma. We realize that congenital anomalies (Cheitlin et al, 1974; Roberts et al, 1982; Taylor et al, 1992b) may produce the clinical pattern of ischemic heart disease. Also, that other pathologic conditions may occlude a coronary artery, e.g., dissecting aneurysm (Silver, 1968; Claudon et al, 1972), emboli (Wenger et al, 1958) or arteritis (Burns et al, 1969) and produce the same effects. However, all of these rare conditions have a dissimilar pathogenic background; so are not discussed further.

CORONARY ARTERY SPASM

The existence of coronary spasm was postulated long ago (Leary, 1935) and proved fact, rather than artifact, by cineangiography of the main subepicardial coronary arteries in ischemic heart disease patients with angina pectoris (Dhurandhar et al, 1972; Oliva et al, 1973; Maseri et al, 1978), or acute myocardial infarction (Cheng et al, 1972; Oliva et al, 1977; Maseri et al, 1978) or in myocardial infarction without coronary disease (Vincent et al, 1983). Contraction bands affecting smooth muscle cells of the tunica media of coronary arteries were proposed as its histologic hallmark (Factor, 1985). However, the diagnosis of spasm postmortem is problematic and its cause still undetermined. In a few instances where it was possible to histologically examine a coronary artery with documented angiographic spasm, the latter occurred in a severely stenosed atherosclerotic vessel. Recently, where focal spasm was induced in patients by ergonovine maleate, small atherosclerotic plaques, undetected angiographically, were demonstrable by intravascular ultrasound (Yamagashi et al, 1994). Furthermore, vasoconstriction or spasm of resistive intramural arterial vessels was postulated to cause ischemia in man (Hellstrom,1982; Pupita et al, 1990; Maseri et al, 1992; Galassi et al, 1994) and was, apparently, demonstrated in the cardiomyopathic Syrian hamster as a cause of focal myocardial necrosis (Factor et al, 1982).

THROMBOTIC CORONARY OCCLUSION

The major cause of coronary occlusion in ischemic heart disease is a luminal thrombus (Fig. 8A,B). Its frequency of occurrence is still debated. Morphologic studies have given a frequency in sudden coronary death (Table 32) from 10-82% with a mean of 29%. A similar range is reported in acute infarct cases. From the earliest reports of myocardial infarction (Hammer, 1878; Herrick, 1912, 1919) the attention of pathologists and clinicians focused on the frequency of the occlusive coronary thrombus with the conclusion that at autopsy in the majority of large, transmural infarcts one is demonstrable (Chandler et al, 1974; Freifeld et al, 1983: transmural 91%, nontransmural 51%). More recently "a fresh, large ($\geq$3000 μm^2) thrombus characterized by its layered organization, aggregates of platelets, fibrin and erythrocytes" was documented histologically in plaques removed by directional atherectomy in 44% of patients with unstable angina or recent (2 weeks) myocardial infarction versus 17% of patients with stable angina (Rosenschein et al, 1994).

By coronary cineangiography, done on 322 patients with acute, Q- wave myocardial infarction, a coronary occlusion was seen in 87% of 126 subjects examined within 4 hours of the onset of their symptoms. In an additional 10% of patients a subtotal occlusion ($\geq$95%) was observed. Similar results were obtained in that study amongst 82 patients evaluated between 4 to 6 hours of onset of their acute infarct (85% and 11% respectively). In contrast, amongst 2 groups each of 57 subjects, one examined between 6 and 12 hours and the other between 12 and 24 hours of infarction, an angiographic total, or subtotal, coronary artery occlusion was observed in 17% and 16% respectively (De Wood et al, 1980). In another study of 341 patients with acute, non-Q-wave, myocardial infarction, 192 had coronary arteriographic studies within 24 hours, 94 between 24 and 72 hours and 55 between 72 hours and 7 days after peak symptoms. Total occlusion of the infarct-related vessel was observed in 26%, 37% and 42% respectively while subtotal occlusion ($\geq$90%) was seen in 34%, 25% and 18% respectively (De Wood et al, 1986). Finally, amongst 59 patients with definite angiographic features of an occlusive thrombus, all of whom subsequently had emergency surgical revascularization, a thrombus was recovered from 88% by intravascular passage of a Fogarty catheter. The thrombi were "consistently situated proximal to the area of stenosis" and were described thus: "the leading edge of each recovered thrombus demonstrated varying quantities of acute inflammatory cells. The number of cells ranged from a few to several hundred per highpower field. The consistent feature of the distal part of every recovered thrombus was a thickened layer of fibrin and platelets. As the sections progressed toward the middle portion of the thrombus, fibrin and platelets became interspersed with red cells, creating a distinct layering effect" (De Wood et al, 1980).

In this context, definition of the terms *thrombus* and *coagulum* is paramount. For instance, in *Dorland's Illustrated Medical Dictionary* (25th Edition, 1974, WB Saunders, Philadelphia) a thrombus is defined as, "An aggregation of blood factors primarily platelets and fibrin with entrapment of cellular elements causing vascular obstruction at the point of its formation" and a coagulum as, "a blood clot formed either in or out of the body." A thrombus is initiated by platelet adhesion at a site of damaged endothelium. Subsequent release of factors from platelets (mainly) or other sites, triggers both further platelet aggregation/adhesion and fibrin deposition. Recurrent platelet aggregation/release/fibrin deposition leads to layers of fibrin-platelet aggregates (Zahn's lines) being formed with or without associated entrapped red cells and polymorphonuclear leukocytes. A thrombus presents in the gross as an opaque, gray-pink mass that is firmly adherent to the vessel wall and not easily removed from it. In contrast, a coagulum maintains the composition of the blood, i.e., is composed mainly of red cells, a few leukocytes, platelets and thin strands of fibrin. Grossly it is a glistening, elastic mass not attached to the vessel wall and easily squeezed from a vessel lumen.

When there is slowing of blood flow, layering of all blood components occurs (Fig. 8D,E). As indicated by Boyd in his pathology text (1965): "It is convenient to consider coagulation and thrombosis separately, although the two are usually inextricably combined. *Coagulation* or *clotting* can occur in the test tube or in the vessels after the blood has ceased to flow, as well as in blood which is still in motion. Its primary constituent is fibrin, in the network of which are entangled the various formed elements of the blood. Chief amongst these are the red cells, so that the clot or coagulum is red and soft, and is referred to as red clot or sometimes (unfortunately) as a red thrombus. A better term is a fibrin or coagulation clot. A *true thrombus*, as we shall see presently, consists primarily of platelets but these are associated with fibrin and a limited number of blood cells. It is correctly described as a white or firm thrombus. If the end result, the clot and the thrombus, may resemble one another, the process by which they are produced are entirely distinct." Because of their entirely different structure one wonders if these two processes may have a similar end result (see below). For sure, the red tail of a white thrombus is caused by stasis of flow in cul de sacs formed at either sides of a firm, adherent thrombus. Therefore this "red tail" or coagulum is an effect of stasis and does not form where flow is present. The claim that in a coronary artery this tail may grow invading functioning distal vessels and thereby increasing ischemia by occluding other branches distal to the thrombotic occlusion is an unproved and improbable hypothesis.

Fate of the Coronary Thrombus

A thrombus undergoes organization by endothelized spaces forming in its substance following platelet contraction and/or by the sprouting into it of capillaries from the vessel wall, the latter accompanied by macrophages and fibroblasts with progressive collagen deposition. Healing ends usually by the occlusive thrombosis becoming a fibrous mass that fills the lumen and may show some recanalization. Mural thrombi undergo a similar process (Fig. 8C).

Postmortem lysis of coronary thrombi, to explain their absence at autopsy, is often advocated. Indeed, spontaneous disappearance of a "coronary occlusion" in vivo is commonly observed by cineangiography. This disappearance is attributed to resolution of vessel wall spasm or to lysis of a thrombus but this may, or may not, be so (see chapter 4). However, the hypothesis that spontaneous reopening of a coronary artery or branch is frequent 6 hours after the onset of symptoms in AMI patients, has been denied recently: Rentrop et al, (1989b) in an angiographic study found spontaneous reflow in an occluded coronary artery within 3-14 hours of the onset of symptoms.

It must be stressed that in experimental occlusion induced by intraluminal coronary thrombosis followed by myocardial infarction, lysis of the thrombus did not occur. Rather, the vessel lumen remained totally occluded in 67% of dogs and partially reopened (75-25% stenosis) in 33% at 17 days (Weisse et al, 1969). Lysis or recanalization of thrombus in this setting is, therefore, a limited and delayed process. Furthermore, in these experiments thrombus formation occurred in a normal coronary artery. In contrast, in man occlusive thrombi are related to atherosclerotic plaques where a reduction of fibrinolytic activity in the wall has been documented experimentally (Myasnikov et al, 1961).

Fate of Coagulum

Subsequent changes in a coagulum, comparable to these described above, are less well known. It seems likely that its completely different structure implies a different fate. It has been stated: "The average atheromatous abscess has been subjected to repeated micro-hemorrhage over a long period and its pultaceous contents is partly haemic in origin" (Morgan, 1956). In hearts excised at transplantation for cardiac failure due to previous myocardial infarct and in which bypass surgery was done long before, we observed some venous grafts, with thickened but not atherosclerotic walls and minor concentric lumen reduction, whose lumen was filled by yellow, toothpaste-like material, easily squeezed from the lumen. Histologically, the graft along its whole course had a lumen totally filled by atheromatous material. This finding suggests that a coagulum rather than undergoing organization like thrombus, after a time may break down and transform into atheromatous-like material giving the false impression of "pultaceous occlusion" following hypothetical rupture of an enormous, undemonstrable atherosclerotic plaque.

NATURAL HISTORY OF COLLATERALS

Postmortem Morphology of Collaterals

In contrast to results obtained by others (Blumgart et al, 1970) the tridimensional coronary casts showed that homo- and intercoronary collaterals normally exist in the human heart (Fig. 10). They are demonstrable at birth and may work in infancy. For example, in cases with an anomalous origin of a coronary artery from the pulmonary artery, left-to-right shunts caused by a pressure gradient between aorta and pulmonary arteries, occur via collaterals. Here the need is to better define the natural history of these vessels in human pathology. Our coronary cast study indicates that in three circumstances homo- and intercoronary collateral vessels increase in size, namely in cardiac hypertrophy, in chronic hypoxic diseases with normal coronary arteries and in the presence of critical coronary stenoses. Only in atrophic hearts with normal coronary arteries are the diameters of collaterals less than normal (Table 42). Therefore, anastomotic channels may enlarge by dilatation and/or hyperplasia of cellular-tissue components of their wall in different conditions, with different causes and with different functional meanings. We have already described the capillary-like composition of the wall of intramural collateral vessels (Fig. 9), with minor and insignificant structural changes occurring even at maximal enlargement, when anastomoses are extramural. We wonder if the term "angiogenesis" used to describe this condition is correct since in the normal myocardium there is no proof of new vessel formation as occurs, for instance, in granulation tissue.

Table 42. Variation of maximal and average diameter of the coronary collateral channels in different states

Status	No cases	Diameter μm	
		Maximum	Average
Normal	(47)	280 (180-350)	200 (150-280)
Atrophy	(13)	240 (150-390)	170 (100-250)
Atrophy + hypoxia	(7)	315 (260-400)	218 (180-280)
Hypertrophy	(21)	350 (200-500)	221 (130-350)
Hypertrophy + hypoxia	(23)	486 (300-700)	304 (180-400)
Hypoxia	(18)	395 (299-395)	249 (180-330)
Mild (<69%) stenosis	(23)	320 (250-425)	209 (165-225)
+ atrophy	(1)	325	225
+ hypertrophy	(16)	318 (250-390)	189 (150-250)
+ hypoxia	(6)	400 (300-600)	242 (200-400)
Severe (70-99%) stenosis	(25)	345 (260-400)	170 (180-200)
+ atrophy	(2)	450 (300-600)	150 (140-160)
+ hypertrophy	(24)	428 (230-1900)	254 (150-460)
+ hypoxia	(8)	461 (300-1000)	307 (150-500)
Occlusion	(35)	685 (350-1250)	347 (200-450)
+ atrophy	(2)	572 (500-650)	350 (300-400)
+ hypertrophy	(55)	729 (290-1690)	413 (125-600)
+ hypoxia	(20)	512 (250-780)	292 (170-550)

Maximum diameter: largest collateral found in single case
Average diameter: average diameter of the larger collaterals (>100μm) found in single cases.

In our opinion the latter rarely forms in the myocardium. We believe that the repair of an infarct or other types of myocardial necrosis is accomplished by collagenization of sarcolemmal tubes without new vessel formation (Baroldi et al, 1975). Granulation tissue does develop along the course of a traumatic wound of the myocardium; then angiogenesis occurs. Implantation of the internal mammary artery or Vineberg's operation, a now abandoned surgical attempt to revascularize the myocardium, provides a good example of a surgical traumatic wound. Following that procedure newly formed anastomotic channels may participate in flow redistribution. However, when implantation is performed in a collateral-dependent zone with a severe stenosis or occlusion of the related coronary artery, the amount and direction of flow in new anastomoses becomes questionable because of competing flow from preexisting collaterals. Lysamine dye injected into the implanted artery remains limited to the immediate area of the implant, unless the main coronary branch is cross-clamped distal to the previous occlusion. In that case, dye distribution approximates the myocardial zone dependent upon the main occluded branch (Mantini et al, 1968). Angiogenesis at the site of an implanted internal mammary artery which provides modest nutritive blood flow to a collateral-dependent region has been considered a model to promote neovascularization suggesting the role of a local angiogenic factor that enhances new collateral formation (Unger et al, 1990). We believe that is a very unlikely phenomenon in normal myocardium. In general, rather than "angiogenesis" or new vessel formation we should speak of *angiohyperplasia,* producing a tridimensional enlargement of preexisting normal vessels by hyperplasia of their wall components, as was observed in both arterial and venous extra- and intramural vessels in hypertrophy of the human heart (Baroldi et al, 1967) and in experimental right ventricular hypertrophy (Farb et al, 1993; Kassab et al, 1993). A similar angiohyperplasia of intramural arterial vessels is seen in chronic hypoxia.

Different mechanisms that trigger collateral angiohyperplasia probably exist. In myocardial hypertrophy/hypoxia an increased oxygen demand (Scheel et al, 1985, 1990) may induce a generalized increase in vessel size by stimulating endothelial growth factors which exist in myocytes (Speir et al, 1988; Weiner et al, 1989; Sasaki et al, 1989; Sasayama et al, 1992). Apparently, collateral growth is also enhanced by heparin (Fujita et al, 1988; Carroll et al, 1993; Quyyumi et al, 1993). The selective increase of satellite collaterals in ischemic heart disease suggests that a pressure gradient, rather than ischemia, is the main stimulus through endothelial cell growth factor (D'Amore et al, 1987) or by increased collateral flow velocity (Flynn et al, 1993). In fact, in the same ischemic zone, a single enlarged collateral may coexist with normal ones; in other words, not all collaterals enlarge in a total ischemic area as they should if ischemia was the main stimulus for their development (Fig. 11C). A fact which contradicts the concept that ischemia, per se, is a collateral-genic factor (Chilian et al, 1990 by experimental microembolization).

Two types of collateral development can be distinguished. One is *diffuse* and affects the whole collateral system associated with an increase in diameter and length of the total intramural system. This is seen in myocardial hypertrophy or hypoxic states. The other is a *regional* development being located and related to a specific lumen reduction of a main arterial vessel (*satellite anastomoses*). Accordingly, two types of collateral function can be considered:

1. In diffuse enlargement, in the presence of normal coronary arteries, the function is mainly *nutritional*, the collaterals forming part of the terminal vascular bed. In fact, their capillary-like structure, their spatial disposition parallel to the plane of contraction of cardiac muscles in a corkscrew arrangement and their systolic flow as demonstrated in cardiac capillaries (Tillmanns et al, 1974), indicate a similar function, i.e., the delivery of nutrient substances to the myocardium. Their enlargement, parallel with other intramural vascular structures, balances an increased demand of the hypertrophied or hypoxic myocardium.

    Inclusion of the collateral system in the terminal vascular bed raises some considerations related to the delivery of oxygen and other substances from capillary to myocell. The geometrical model of one capillary to one cell (Wearn, 1928) or of four equally spaced capillaries per myocell (Ludwig, 1971) should be reconsidered in pathologic states. In reality we deal with a more extensive terminal network that includes collateral vessels and surrounds each myocell in all directions. This complex terminal system seems more appropriate in the face of a wide range of metabolic demands, even in markedly hypertrophied hearts. The lack of relation between infarct size and heart weight speaks against the supposed relative ischemia of hypertrophied myocardium, particularly in cor pulmonale (Baroldi, 1971a).

2. *Redistribution* of nutritional flow is a second function of collaterals in the presence of a critical coronary obstruction (satellite anastomoses). The satellite pattern may be ill-defined in hearts with multiple severe obstructions and previous infarcts. Satellite collaterals in the presence of a functional stenosis appear to supply nutritional blood to the dependent ischemic territory (Fig. 10).

A fact to stress is the high variability of the anastomotic index in the different groups of hearts examined in the plastic cast study (Table 42). Another is the different patterns of collateralization found in the presence of coronary obstruction of comparable location and degree. For example, occlusion at the same site of a main coronary artery may be "compensated" by a relatively few, very enlarged anastomoses, easily seen by cineangiography, or by many, relatively small (100-300 μm), anastomoses that are not, or are poorly demonstrated by cineangiography. Despite assertions that angiographic techniques permit the imaging of intramural vessels of 100 μm diameter (Gensini et al, 1969), we note in reality, that a comparison between plastic casts of coronary arteries and cineangiographic images of them clearly shows a difference in their number and size demonstrated by these techniques.

Two factors may be responsible for the high variability of collateral patterns seen in ischemic heart disease either in vivo or postmortem. The first is a progression of atherosclerosis in the whole extramural coronary system. Adjustment to flow redistribution and related anatomical changes would depend on the chronological development and location of plaques in different coronary arteries or their branches.

The second factor would be infarct necrosis. In the latter condition and proportionate to infarct size, postmortem coronary injection of radiopaque or plastic material fails to fill intramural vessels in an infarcted zone. As described later, stretching and compression of infarcted myocardium by intraventricular pressure and subsequent thrombosis of intramural vessels within necrotic tissue lead to an intramural "*avascular area*" where only extramural branches can be seen (Fig. 11). In a healed infarct the histologic picture is of hyaline, dense and avascular connective tissue, sometimes crossed and often surrounded by giant capillaries (*angiomatous plexus*). The latter are, in fact, already visible during repair (Fig. 12). The disappearance of all intramural arterial vessels, including collaterals, suggests that surviving anastomoses may further enlarge since the pressure gradient between the stenosed, infarct-related artery and adjacent vascular territories is still active. It is likely that highly enlarged collaterals are those seen by angiography.

A last comment relates to the *plaque satellite anastomotic network* (Fig. 13) in advanced plaque. Its highly variable morphology is likely due to the chronological interaction between plaque growth/vascularization and redistribution of flow through other satellite intramural collaterals.

Angiographic Morphology of Collaterals

In many angiographic studies of patients undergoing aortocoronary bypass grafting or angioplasty or intracoronary thrombolysis following an acute myocardial infarction, the presence of collaterals has been investigated and correlated with other functional variables. In these an increased frequency of collaterals was seen related to the number of main vessels with severe stenoses (>50%); however, both the number of stenoses and the presence or absence of collaterals did not correlate with hemodynamic abnormalities, e.g., left ventricular end-diastolic pressure and cardiac index. Ventriculographic alterations correlated with an increasing number of diseased vessels but not with the presence of collaterals, suggesting the lack of their protection (Helfant et al, 1970; Bodenheimer et al, 1977). A flow restriction was observed in collateral dependent myocardium in patients with complete occlusion of the left anterior descending artery (Arani et al, 1984). In patients undergoing aortocoronary bypass grafting total coronary artery occlusion associated with collaterals showed hemodynamic changes, i.e., poststenotic coronary pressure and graft flow hyperemia that simulated those of a 90% coronary stenosis without collaterals. On the other hand, left ventricular asynergy increased with the severity of coronary obstruction without relation to angiographically significant collaterals (63% of hypo- or akinetic wall segments in chronic coronary occlusion with collaterals versus 45% with <80% stenosis, 52% with 80-90% stenosis and 57% with 91-99% stenosis without collaterals; Flameng et al, 1978).

Patients with angina pectoris and persistent occlusion of a major coronary artery but without previous myocardial infarction have, by positron emission tomography, a similar regional myocardial blood flow and both oxidative metabolism and glucose uptake in collateral-dependent and remote myocardial segments with normal wall motion. In contrast, a lessened myocardial blood flow, reduced oxidative metabolism and higher glucose uptake were observed in dysfunctioning collateral-dependent myocardial segments compared to normal, remote, ones. However, when collateral-dependent segments with and without abnormal wall motion were compared, no differences in blood flow were found. After intravenous dipyridamole, collateral-dependent myocardial blood flow greatly increased in segments with normal wall motion, while the increase was minimal if associated with asynergy. A functional follow-up in patients undergoing percutaneous transluminal coronary angioplasty (8 cases) or coronary artery bypass surgery (4 cases) revealed adequate revascularization in 11, reocclusion in 1 after successful angioplasty. In all, including the reoccluded subject, regional wall motion improved (Vanoverschelde et al, 1993). In another positron emission tomography study, patients with stable exertional angina, normal ventricular function and chronic occlusion of a major extramural artery, opacified via intramyocardial collateral flow, myocardial blood flow at rest equaled that in normal volunteers in areas of normal myocardium and in myocardial collateral-perfused areas of the patients. However, following dipyridamole the increased flow in collateral-perfused areas was only one half that in normal areas (McFalls et al, 1993).

In another clinical analysis most patients with severe coronary stenosis had collateral channel filling improved within 60-90 seconds of angioplasty after a sudden coronary balloon occlusion (Rentrop et al, 1985). The left ventricular function and clinical outcome after abrupt coronary closure depended upon the location of the coronary artery obstruction and degree of collateral flow (Rentrop et al, 1988). A study of patients with a myocardial infarction 2 days to 5 weeks earlier who developed asynergic wall motion, revealed that 78% of them had improved ventricular function when angioplasty was successful, in contrast to 11% with unsuccessful angioplasty. This improvement correlated with the percentage of infarct bed (>50%) supplied by collateral flow, assessed by myocardial contrast echocardiography and was independent of the time between infarction and angioplasty. Myocardium remains viable for a prolonged period and its viability seems associated with the presence of collaterals (Sabia et al, 1992). On the other hand, repetitive coronary occlusion, e.g., five successive prolonged inflations at angioplasty in patients with chronic angina and an isolated critical (≥70%) stenosis of the left anterior descending coronary branch and normal left ventricular function induced a progressive adaptation to myocardial ischemia with reduction of symptoms and of ischemic ECG changes by recruiting collateral channels, evaluated by ipsilateral and contralateral injection of contrast medium and hemodynamically by occlusion pressure, suggesting an underlying mechanism of myocardial ischemic preconditioning (Cribier et al, 1992). A concept reported previously by Deutsch et al (1990).

The many clinical studies cited and numerous editorials (Cohen,1978; Gregg et al, 1980; Topol et al, 1991; Sasayama et al, 1992) emphasize uncertainties about the functional role of coronary collaterals in ischemic heart disease. In fact, other papers document the role of preexisting collaterals in preventing postinfarct left ventricular aneurysm formation (Forman et al, 1986; Habib et al, 1991) despite their inability to improve ventricular function (Hirai et al, 1989). Amongst patients with unsuccessful thrombolysis, in the presence of collateral vessels at the onset of a myocardial infarct, other authors found a limitation of infarct size as assessed enzymatically (Habib et al, 1991) and improved ventricular function determined by left ventricular ejection fraction (Williams et al, 1976; Nohara et al, 1983; Rogers et al, 1984; Schwartz et al, 1985; Saito et al, 1985; Habib et al, 1991). Such improved ventricular function was also observed after late thrombolytic therapy, within 12 hours, but not with nitroglycerin intracoronary infusion (Rentrop et al, 1989a). Keep in mind that successful recanalization by intracoronary thrombolysis in acute infarct patients without demonstrable collaterals did not improve left ventricular function (Rogers et al, 1984; Saito et al, 1985).

Experimental Studies on Collaterals

Data from experiments help understand the natural history of collaterals (Gregg, 1974). After an abrupt occlusion of a normal coronary artery in a dog, collateral indices such as coronary pressure distal to occlusion and collateral flow into the ischemic area, show a variable, small collateral circulation ranging from 10-32% of normal aortic blood pressure and coronary inflow for minutes to hours. During the first 24 hours following occlusion subendocardial collateral flow increases and often doubles. Gradual coronary stenosis, on the other hand, induces a large increase in collateral indices without evidence of myocardial damage. The release of a coronary occlusion that lasted from 7-10 days caused an immediate decline in this increased collateral function; it reached preocclusion levels within 3 to 24 hours. Reocclusion of the same coronary vessel 2 months later, rapidly reestablished collateral flow at its previous high values (Khouri et al, 1971; Gregg, 1980).

This long list of postmortem, clinical and experimental data help outline the natural history of collaterals in ischemic heart disease/sudden death. They exist but their function is controversial. This will serve as background for a discussion on their significance (see chapter 4).

NATURAL HISTORY OF MYOCARDIAL CELL NECROSIS

Different forms of myocardial cell necrosis are observed in ischemic heart disease (see above). A basic question is whether all are related to ischemia or each has a distinct cause and pathogenic mechanism. This must be resolved if we wish to understand the natural history of different clinical patterns in ischemic heart disease and how they cause death. The rationale to correctly discriminate between different types of myonecrosis is their correlation with myocardial cell function. This will be discussed after a review of that cell's functional anatomy.

FUNCTIONAL ANATOMY OF THE MYOCARDIAL CELL

Myocardial cells (or myocells) are the functional units of heart muscle. Grossly they form four main muscle bundles, two internal circumferential ones and two external helicoidal ones, each anchored to the fibrous framework of the heart located about valves and large vessels. This architectural structure allows twisting/shortening contractions of the myocardium with optimal blood ejection. The heart muscle is not an anatomical syncytium because at its extremities each myocell, a cylindric structure 50-100 μm long and 10-20 μm wide, is separated by, and connected with, adjacent myocells by intercalated discs. Nevertheless, if individual cells are not a syncytium anatomically, heart muscle can at least be defined as a functional syncytium capable of rhythmic contraction/relaxation cycles. The function of the normal cardiac pump is achieved by contraction of all myocells coordinated by neurogenic impulses via the conduction system, regulated by intramyocardial nervous reflexes. It begins at the third week of fetal life and when it stops life usually ends. Cessation of contractile function is frequently a cause of death.

The contractile apparatus of any single myocell is formed by a bundle of cylindric myofibrils each one subdivided into 20-50 subunits *(sarcomeres)* separated by thin *Z lines*. A sarcomere constitutes the basic functional unit and is constructed for repetitive contraction/

relaxation cycles. It is formed by two centrally separated sets of *thin* or *actin filaments* (1-μm long) implanted on two limiting Z lines. Parallel to and between the thin filaments are thick *L-meromyosin filaments* (1.5 μm long) located in the central part of the sarcomere. Thick filaments are not attached to Z lines. Thin and thick filaments have lateral, corresponding digitations, tropomyosin-troponin and H-meromyosin respectively, which are the active sites of the biochemical *hinge* which regulates contraction/relaxation. This is achieved by a back-and-forth movement of thin filaments which penetrate the other half of the sarcomere by "sliding" on the thick filaments (*sliding theory*). In diastole the tropomyosin-troponin complex inhibits contraction. The latter is reestablished by Ca^{++} binding to troponin. Therefore, the contraction/relaxation cycle is obtained by to-and-fro rhythmic pumping of Ca^{++} from its stores in the sarcoplasmic reticulum to myofibrils and vice versa.

All myofibrils are in a registered order and give the myocell its characteristic regular cross-striations. However, cross-striations vary according to cell function. In relaxation sarcomere length is normally 2.4 μm while in contraction it is 1.5 μm. The systolic length of a sarcomere ranges from 1.86-1.95 μm and the diastolic length from 2.05-2.15 μm. The length giving maximal active tension, in relationship to the Starling phenomenon, has been calculated at 2.20-2.35 μm (end-diastolic reserve; Spiro et al, 1968).

Different aspects of the sarcomere are revealed by electron microscopy during various phases of contraction and relaxation. In relaxation two clear *I bands,* formed only by thin filaments, are visible at both sides of a Z line. Internal to the I bands are two more dense *S bands*, which include both actin and myosin filaments. In cross section, one thick myosin filament is encircled by six thin actin filaments arrayed in hexagonal order. Other bands, formed only by myosin filaments, are visible in the central part of the sarcomere. They constitute the *H-L-M complex.* It consists of a unique darker band in the center with two L bands and two H bands in lateral positions. Together the H-L-M complex and the S bands are defined as the *A band.* In normal maximal contraction, I and H bands disappear because of the total penetration of thin filaments on one side of the sarcomere into the other; in cross section their number is doubled. The A band remains formed by the S and L-M bands plus the C_m *(maximal contraction) band*, which includes both actin and myosin filaments. The different types of bands and Z lines are clearly defined by electron microscopy. With light microscopy and high magnification, very thin Z lines may be recognized between two adjacent clear, I bands when the myocell is relaxed. In contrast, Z lines become distinct in hypercontracted myofibers because of a drastic increase in their thickness.

Different Forms of Myocardial Damage Related to Myocell Function

The myocardial cell may stop functioning in irreversible relaxation, in contraction, or may progressively lose its force and velocity. Each situation produces a different morphologic form of irreversible myocardial damage.

Atonic Death in Irreversible Relaxation

This type of myocardial necrosis (*infarct necrosis*) is observed when myocells lose their capability to contract, becoming passive and extensible elements (Fig. 14). This loss of contraction both occurs and can be seen within a few seconds of experimentally occluding a dog's coronary artery (Tennant et al, 1935, 1936; Jennings, 1969). The acutely ischemic myocardium becomes cyanosed and because of intraventricular pressure shows a paradoxical, systolic bulging. The histologic counterpart of this flaccid paralysis (with stretching and reduction in thickness of the infarcted wall) is a thinning of the mildly eosinophilic necrotic myocells with elongation of sarcomeres and nuclei. These changes are visible within 1 hour of experimental coronary artery occlusion (Hort, 1968; Baroldi et al, 1977).

Other histologic changes in chronological sequence are seen in both experimental animal and man:

1. A centripetal polymorphonuclear leukocytic (PMN) infiltration from the periphery of the infarct occurs within 6 to 8 hours with minimal exudate of edema fluid, fibrin and red cells. PMNs increase in number during the next 24 hours and disappear by lysis within the first week of onset, without evident destruction of necrotic myocells. Large infarcts may show a central area where the sequence of changes to be described does not occur. Rather, the mildly eosinophilic, stretched, dead myofibers persist. This is due to blockage of PMN penetration caused by maximal stretching of the central part of the dead tissue. Furthermore, if a marked PMN infiltration develops at the edge of sequestered, dead myocardium, the overall appearance may resemble an abscess with myocell destruction.

2. *Fibrin/platelet thrombotic occlusion* of intramural vessels included in the infarcted zone occurs parallel to, but not before the PMN infiltration.

3. The *healing process,* which starts 1 week after infarction, begins at the periphery by macrophagic digestion of necrotic material within sarcolemmal tubes (Fig. 15A) and is followed by progressive collagenization. In contrast to other authors (Mallory et al, 1939), we believe the latter occurs without a granulation tissue response (Baroldi et al, 1975).

Intimal obstructive thickening of small arteries is seen at the periphery of the early healing zone (Baroldi, 1967).

Three further findings and three comments complete histologic observations in this type of necrosis. First, the registered order of sarcomeres may be maintained for a long time in remnants of dead myocells in healed infarcts (>30 days) and if entrapped in scar (Fig. 15B). Second, the lack of filling by postmortem injection of intramural arterial vessels is noticeable in an acute infarct (*avascular area*, see above). Third, this type of necrosis usually presents as one focus. It may affect the subendocardial zone or a greater width of the ventricular wall and can be transmural. Its size ranges from less than 10% to more than 50% of left ventricular mass. Very rarely it presents as small multiple foci in the subendocardium. We would like to comment about the designation "coagulation necrosis" given this form of necrosis, despite the lack of coagulation of structures in its various phases. The more explicit term *infarct necrosis* seems more appropriate. Another comment relates to the hemorrhagic nature of infarct necrosis seen after fibrinolytic therapy (Fujiwara et al, 1986). Rarely, a myocardial infarct may be hemorrhagic, e.g., when associated with wall rupture (Oliva et al, 1993) or therapeutic procedures. A last comment concerns "wavy fibers," i.e., undulated myocardial fibers proposed as an early sign of myocardial ischemia (Bouchardy et al, 1971-72). When found, their lack of specificity does not permit, per se, a diagnosis of ischemia. In fact, waviness of normal myocells is usually observed around hypercontracted myocardial fibers (see below).

TETANIC DEATH IN IRREVERSIBLE CONTRACTION

This form of myocardial necrosis presents an opposite pattern to infarct necrosis. Here the myocell is unable to relax and its function arrests in contraction, or more precisely in hypercontraction because of an extreme reduction in sarcomere length, much less than 1.5 μm calculated for normal contraction.

Several different morphologies may result from hypercontraction:

Coagulative myocytolysis or Zenker necrosis

This lesion has also been defined as anomalous contraction bands (Herdson et al, 1975); focal myocytolysis (Schlesinger et al, 1955); focal myocarditis with myofibrillar degeneration (Szakacs et al, 1958); infarct-like myocardial necrosis (Rona et al, 1959); myocytolysis with major contraction bands (Bloom et al, 1969); myofibrillar degeneration (Reichenbach et al, 1970) and necrosis with contraction bands (Ferrans et al, 1975). We prefer the term *myocytolysis* adding the adjective *coagulative* to emphasize the coagulation of contractile proteins seen. Alternatively, the term *Zenker necrosis* used in the past for a similar change described in skeletal muscle (Adam, 1975), suffices.

This lesion (Fig. 16), which is characteristic of, and the only one found in, catecholamine cardiotoxicity (Todd et al, 1985a), is also detected in many other pathologic conditions in man, e.g., pheochromocytoma, transplanted heart, thrombotic thrombocytopenic purpura, "stone heart," ischemic heart disease, electrocution, malignant hyperthermia, scleroderma, etc. and in experimental models associated with catecholamine infusion, stellate ganglion stimulation, electric shock, magnesium deficiency, psychological stress, etc. (Baroldi, 1991b).

The first change is a hypercontraction of the whole myocell with markedly thickened Z lines and extremely short sarcomeres. Myocells become intensely eosinophilic and their sarcoplasm subsequently fragments into irregular total or partial transverse acidophilic bands or present a diffuse granular appearance. These deeply staining cytoplasmic bands in hematoxylin and eosin sections alternate with clear, empty spaces or with spaces filled by small dark granules. Ultrastructurally, a transverse band appears as a small group of hypercontracted sarcomeres with highly thickened Z lines or as amorphous, darkly electron dense material, likely the result of coagulation of contractile proteins. The clear spaces are filled by normal or slightly swollen mitochondria containing dense, fine granules and occasionally showing rupture of their cristae. The sarcotubular system is totally disrupted while the basement membrane is essentially intact; only occasionally are interruptions seen in its continuity. Folding of the sarcolemma expresses the hypercontractile state of sarcomeres. Glycogen deposits disappear without evidence of intracellular or interstitial edema. There is no damage to blood vessels hence no associated hemorrhage with the myocell necrosis nor are platelet aggregates or platelet/fibrin thrombi found. (Todd et al, 1985). It seems likely that the degree of fragmentation of the rigid, inextensible myocells in irreversible hypercontraction is a consequence of the mechanical action of normal contracting myocardium around them.

The acute lesion described above is detectable in experimental conditions within 15 minutes of an intravenous infusion of norepinephrine or isoproterenol. It may involve a single myocell among thousands of normal ones, foci of a few myocells or large zones of myocardium. The degree of involvement in such experiments is dose-dependent and the lesion plurifocal.

This damage does not elicite a PMN leukocyte infiltration. Later, monocytes appear to digest necrotic material within sarcolemmal tubes leading to an *alveolar* pattern (Schlesinger's original "myocytolysis") followed by progressive collapse and collagenization by activation of interstitial cells. This occurs in the affected areas without angiogenesis, i.e., evident granulation tissue formation. We believe this repair process is identical to that seen in infarct necrosis but have no exact idea of its speed in these generally smaller lesions.

Paradiscal contraction band

This myocellular lesion may be found in all conditions where coagulative myocytolysis occurs (Fig. 17). It presents a unique band of less than 15 hypercontracted sarcomeres adjacent to an intercalated disc. The remaining part of the myocell is normal. The band, with related scalloped sarcolemma, shows two typical ultrastructural aspects. One is a *clear paradiscal contraction band* formed by extremely shortened sarcomeres closely packed together with ill-defined, often fragmented, thin Z lines while myofilaments are visible without evidence of rhexis. All mitochondria seem squeezed together in the normal portion of the myocell. Another aspect is an increased electron density of different degrees of intensity, from almost clear to deeply dark, that crosses the whole paradiscal band. These dark bands are also visible histologically.

A paradiscal band is often observed at both sides of an intercalated disc and has generally a greater diameter than the other, normal portion of the myocell. Adjacent normal myocells show a wavy disposition (Fig. 18C), possibly induced by the hypercontracted myocell. In cross section, myocells affected by paradiscal lesions show large, deeply eosinophilic elements with a spoked-wheel aspect on phosphotungstic acid and hematoxylin stain.

We believe paradiscal contraction bands are the equivalent of *zonal lesions* described in hemorrhagic shock (Martin et al, 1963,1966). They are prevented by beta-blocking agents (Entman et al, 1965). The paradiscal band is observed within 5 minutes of intravenous catecholamine infusion. Its subsequent evolution is not known. Not seen at subsequent examination six days after onset, it may be a reversible lesion. Furthermore, we do not know if clear and dark bands are two separate entities or sequential aspects of the same lesion. Since, in general, hypercontraction is characterized by thickened Z lines plus very short sarcomeres leading to a coagulated dark band, one may speculate that the dark aspect is the beginning of a hypercontracted paradiscal lesion while the clear one could be related to a rebuilding of normal structure. The absence of fragmentation of myofibrils in this type of band is likely due to its paradiscal location at the extremity of an otherwise normally functioning myocell. On the other hand, segmental hypercontraction within a cell may lead to stretching and rhexis of adjacent nonhypercontracted sarcomeres; a finding often observed between two myocells in line, one hypercontracted and the other hyperdistended.

Reflow necrosis

Frequently diagnosed as "infarct necrosis" clinically, *reflow necrosis* seems related to increased flow following ischemia or anoxia in which catecholamines (Raab, 1970) and ionic calcium may have an important role. It may be defined as coagulative myocytolysis associated with hemorrhage. One notes that after temporary hypocalcemia, restoration to normocalcemia induces myocardial contraction band lesions (*Ca++ paradox phenomenon*, Zimmerman et al, 1967; Hearse et al, 1978). We note that perfusion with Ca++ free blood following coronary occlusion protects the dependent myocardium (Ashrof et al, 1978).

Reflow necrosis is found in patients subject to long-lasting resuscitative attempts or following heart surgery (Lie et al, 1978) and in experimental temporary coronary occlusion. It may be extensive, involve the inner half of the left ventricle and interventricular septum and be associated with massive hemorrhage producing *concentric hemorrhagic necrosis* (Gottlieb et al, 1977). There is also intramyocardial vessel wall damage with luminal platelet aggregates plus a scanty PMN leukocyte exudate. In the experimental situation, reflow induces malignant arrhythmias (Reimer et al, 1977). Both the pathological changes and arrhythmias can be prevented in different ways, e.g., hypothermia and by different chemical substances, including beta-blockers (Reimer et al, 1976).

Contraction bands at the cut edges of living myocardium

We note that at a site of myocardial biopsy or along the cut edges of hearts excised at transplantation, living myocells retract with sarcoplasmic band formation (Fig. 18). The depth of this hypercontracted margin is between 0.2 and 0.5 mm (Todd et al, 1985) and the pattern consists of hypercontracted sarcomeres with thickened Z lines, forming transverse and parallel bands without evidence of myofibrillar disruption. Such traumatic changes, also obvious in small endomyocardial biopsy samples are not caused by ischemia.

FAILING DEATH OF MYOCELLS OR PROGRESSIVE LOSS OF FUNCTION

In this pattern and in contrast with previous types of myonecrosis, the cell maintains its function with a gradually reduced capacity to contract ending in an insufficient heart. The histologic marker is a progressive loss of myofibrils associated with intracellular edema and with different degrees of damage from mild vacuolization (moth-eaten pattern) to total disappearance of myofibrils (Fig. 19). This produces an alveolar pattern but, in contrast to other forms of myonecrosis mentioned above, the alveolar pattern lacks macrophages or any other cell reaction. The impression is a colliquation or washout of myofibrils that leaves a sarcolemmal sheath with a clear alveolar appearance (*colliquative myocytolysis*) in a cytoplasm at most filled by edema and/or packed small granules (mitochondria).

Each of the three functional forms of myocardial damage described above has a distinct structural and biochemical nature. In irreversible relaxation intracellular acidosis displaces Ca++ from troponin (loss of contraction; Katz 1971/1972, 1988; Opie, 1993). During irreversible hypercontraction intracellular alkalosis induces a rapid loss of ATP with a lack of energy to remove Ca^{++} from troponin (Meerson, 1969) and/or a massive intracellular influx of Ca^{++} (Fleckenstein et al, 1975) from increased membrane permeability. This leads, by activation of myofibrillar ATPase, to contraction and ATP consumption. In the failing death of myocells the sarcotubular system and mitochondria have a reduced capacity to bind Ca^{++} (Bing et al, 1974).

The presence and frequency of all three types of myonecrosis in the natural history of ischemic heart disease has been reported above (Table 2). We recall that at the outer and lateral edges of infarct necrosis a rim of coagulative myocytolysis of variable width is always found. A change referred to in an early pathological report on myocardial infarcts (Mallory et al, 1939) and more recently reconfirmed (Freifeld et al, 1983) in man and experimental animals (Shen et al, 1971). Furthermore, isolated or confluent foci of coagulative myocytolysis are visible in noninfarcted zones around the infarct and in other noninfarcted cardiac regions in 90% of AMI cases (Baroldi et al, 1974; Silver et al, 1980). Finally, in 40% of the latter, particularly in chronic ischemic heart disease cases with extensive myocardial fibrosis, colliquative myocytolysis is observed in subendocardial and perivascular myocells. In general, these areas are not affected by infarct necrosis.

In sudden and unexpected death cases, coagulative myocytolysis is the unique acute myocardial lesion in 72% of cases and is present in all such subjects with demonstrated infarct necrosis. In contrast colliquative myocytolysis was found in only 8% of cases, mainly associated with severe myocardial fibrosis (Baroldi et al, 1979).

REVERSIBLE VS. IRREVERSIBLE MYOCARDIAL DAMAGE IN RELATION TO DYSFUNCTION

Ischemic heart disease causes temporary or permanent and regional or global heart muscle dysfunction (*asynergy* or *dissynergy*). Three main patterns are distinguished viz *hypokinesis,* i.e., reduction of contractility, *akinesis,* i.e., absence of contraction and *dyskinesis,* i.e., absence of contraction plus paradoxical systolic bulging. Radionucleide angiography and echocardiography are essential to establish cardiac wall asynergy in life. Echocardiography during dobutamine infusion can distinguish between permanent and temporary asynergic areas (Pierard et al, 1990). Of 314 akinetic segments in 33 chronic ischemic heart disease patients, 58% became normokinetic and 7% hypokinetic after venous bypass surgery. Dobutamine infusion was able to predict improvement in 198 of the 205 segments that recovered function after surgery (La Canna et al, 1994).

However, a need to establish the structural nature of cardiac dysfunction, even in the normal myocardium of ischemic patients (Uren et al, 1993), is paramount, particularly because two different types of viable, but noncontracting, myocardium have been proposed. They are:

stunned myocardium, which occurs following reflow after a transient episode of ischemia produced by experimental temporary coronary occlusion and needs hours, days or weeks before contraction is restored (Braunwald et al, 1982; Ellis et al, 1983; Schwaiger et al, 1985; Stahl et al, 1987; Manyani et al, 1988; Gropel et al, 1990; Kloner et al, 1990; Moore et al, 1990; Taylor et al, 1992a) and *hibernating myocardium* defined as "a state of persistently impaired myocardial and left ventricular function at rest due to reduced coronary blood flow that can be partially or completely restored to normal if the myocardial oxygen supply/demand relationship is favorably altered either by improving blood flow and/or reducing demand" (Rahimtoola, 1989). In other words, in *chronic ischemia* the myocardium stops contracting teleologically, to save its structure ("smart heart"), ready to contract again as soon as ischemia is alleviated. Less clear, according to definition, is how an already hibernating myocardium can reduce its demands and return to function.

These two dysfunctional patterns (Bollietal, 1988; Bonor et al, 1990) with an apparent diverging pathogenesis, i.e., reflow shortly after nonnecrotic, acute ischemia in stunning, and nonnecrotic chronic ischemia in hibernation, seem not to produce histologic signs or minimal and reversible ultrastructural changes affecting mitochondria in experimental stunned myocardium after 15 minutes of coronary occlusion (Kloner et al, 1989). By repetitive, brief coronary occlusions stunning increases with an increasing number of occlusions ("sensitization"; Schroder et al, 1988) and there is relaxation of muscle fibers (wide I bands), margination of nuclear chromatin, glycogen depletion, intra-and extracellular edema and marked alteration of collagen matrix components (cable, weaves, struts: Zhao et al, 1987).

Histologic and ultrastructural findings in transmural biopsies from dysfunctioning collateral-dependent areas in chronic angina patients with severe stenosis or old occlusion of one or more coronary arteries, with or without an old infarct, demonstrate cellular swelling, loss of myofibrillar content and glycogen accumulation (Flameng et al, 1987; Vanovershelde et al, 1993; Borgers et al, 1993). These changes, similar to those described above as colliquative myocytolysis were considered characteristic of hibernating myocardium and caused by repeated episodes of ischemia and not by chronic hypoperfusion (Vanovershelde et al, 1993). Interpreted as reversible "dedifferentiation" with "partial to complete loss of sarcomeres, sarcoplasmic reticulum, T tubules and abundant plaques of glycogen, strands of rough endoplasmic reticulum, lots of minimitochondria and a tortuous nucleus" rather than degenerative changes, the delayed functional recovery was imputed to slow resynthesis of the contractile apparatus (Borgers et al, 1993). On the other hand, in patients with chronic ischemic heart disease and dilated cardiomyopathy undergoing heart transplantation, myocardial blood flow was similarly impaired in fibrotic and viable myocardium.

This suggested that mechanisms other than myocardial fibrosis and coronary lesions determine blood flow impairment in end stage heart failure (Parodi et al, 1993).

In our definition of the three functional forms of myonecrosis early changes were hyperdistension with enlarged I bands and normal Z lines in infarct necrosis; hypercontraction (very short sarcomeres with markedly thickened Z lines) in Zenker necrosis and progressive myofibril disappearance in colliquative myocytolysis. At present there is no way of establishing if the early stages of these changes are reversible or not. For example, in the first the disconnected interdigitations between thick and thin filaments might be reconnected: in the second, thickened Z lines represent an agglomeration of contractile proteins which might revert to normal. If so, the sliding theory of contraction should include the concept of a reversible "rolling up" of filaments at the Z line level; or if this is not the case, thickened Z lines should be an irreversible sign of damage. In the third lesion the cause of failure could stop with a rebuilding of myofibrils.

At present too, there is no way of structurally recognizing stunned or hibernating myocells or to relate those function changes to the ones described in previous paragraphs. On the other hand, when asynergic zones are matched histologically (Table 43), false-positive, i.e., asynergy with "normal" noncontracting myocardium and false-negative, i.e., myocardial "necrosis," even transmural, without asynergic segments were shown (Cabin et al, 1987). The apparent contradiction of a lack of asynergy associated with transmural necrosis can be explained by the definition given (transmural equals 75% of wall thickness). Perhaps, further quantitative studies are needed to establish the contractile status and type/age of the eventual, associated myocardial lesions. Is the stunned myocardium related to hypercontraction while hibernating myocardium is related to hyperdistension as suggested by functional changes in these two types of damage?

OTHER MORPHOLOGIC VARIABLES IN THE NATURAL HISTORY OF SUDDEN DEATH AND ISCHEMIC HEART DISEASE

We have outlined the pathological background of ischemic heart disease. In referring to personal data and that in the literature, other structural changes have been mentioned and discussed. For instance, platelet aggregates, formed in situ or embolized to intramural vessels or small vessel disease in the context of the various patterns of ischemic heart disease.

Another factor deserving comment is the PMN leukocyte reaction in the early phase of infarct necrosis. The claim is that an increased influx of neutrophils follows reinstitution of flow into an ischemic area by thrombolysis, surgical by-pass or angioplasty. In this condition the striking leukotactic stimulus determines entrapment of these elements

Table 43. Myocardial asynergy versus structural damage

Authors		Disease	Method	Cases No	Segments No (%)	False-positive normal myoc.		False-negative myoc. necrosis	
						Hypokinesis	Akin/Dyskin	Transmural	Nontrans.
Cabin	1987	Acute infarct	RA/A	23	228 (100)	27(12)	6(3)	11(5)	34(15)
Sinusas	1984	Chronic IHD (48) Valvular Cpt (3) Dilated Cmp (4)	RA/A	55	372 (100)	–	35(9)	61(16)	–
Ideker	1978	Chronic IHD	Vq/A	24	72 (100)	–	8(11)	2(3)	–
Hutchins	1977	Chronic IHD (24) Valvular Cpt (4)	V/A	28	140 (100)	56(40)	16(11)	–	1(1)
Stinson	1977	Chronic IHD	V/B	110	110 (100)	12(11)	4(4)	–	15(14)
Bodenheimer	1976	Chronic IHD	V/B	25	29 (100)	11(38)	–	–	–

RA, radionucleide angiography; V, ventriculography; q, quantitative; A, autopsy; B, biopsy
False-positive: asynergy + normal myocardium
False-negative: myocardial necrosis + normal contraction

in microvessels. The effect is a mechanical obstruction of the latter and/or release of vasoconstrictive substances which increase ischemia and/or products toxic to the endothelium. Increased permeability by specific interactions between adhesion protein molecules and the plasma membrane of myocytes; (Engler et al, 1986; Dreyer et al, 1991; Entman et al, 1991), results in a "no-reflow phenomenon." Experimentally, infarct size was reduced by selective inhibition of neutrophil cytotoxic activity without affecting neutrophil migration into injured myocardium (Amsterdam et al, 1993). However, neutrophil depletion did not protect from reperfusion damage (Carlson et al, 1989).

CLINICAL TYPES OF SUDDEN CARDIAC ARREST

Several studies investigated clinical signs in patients at risk of sudden death (Hagstrom et al, 1964; Kannel et al, 1975, 1985; Hammermeister et al, 1977; Hinkle et al, 1977; Vismara et al, 1977; Hamer et al, 1982). A last variable to be considered is the different types of cardiac arrest. From a clinical standpoint (Fisch et al, 1985; Surawicz, 1985) the following electrocardiographic morphologies associated with sudden death are recognized: (1) ventricular fibrillation as an end result of malignant arrhythmia; (2) asystole secondary to neurally-mediated bradycardia/hypotension (Milstein et al, 1989) or progressive reduction of the force/velocity of contraction; (3) electromechanical dissociation (Fozzard et al, 1985), i.e., loss of mechanical function such as pulse, blood pressure, heart sounds and consciousness despite a normal electrocardiogram; a pattern which, in general, ends in asystole. In this last condition no other explanation, e.g., pulmonary embolism or heart rupture with pericardial tamponade, can be found at autopsy (Hackel et al, 1993).

In most ischemic heart disease patients and in subjects dying a sudden and unexpected coronary death, ventricular fibrillation is the most frequent mechanism of cardiac arrest. Among the many predisposing factors which may precipitate this arrhythmia (Gradman et al, 1977; Pool et al, 1978; Proust et al, 1981; Pratt et al, 1983), for example, enlarged heart, mitral valve prolapse, myocarditis, circadian patterns (Peters et al, 1994), psychologic factors (Engel, 1971), catecholamines or sympathetic overactivity; ischemia, particularly induced by coronary plaque rupture and thrombosis predominates (Patterson et al, 1982; Willich et al, 1993).

In two clinical studies the type and nature of cardiac arrest were investigated in a selected population of ischemic heart disease patients. The first was a follow-up of successfully defibrillated people who had sudden cardiac arrest out-of-hospital. Amongst 305 subjects, 19% subsequently developed a transmural myocardial infarction while 42% had ST and T wave changes. Seventy-one had no appreciable ECG alterations during post-resuscitation hospitalization. In 38% of cases lactate dehydrogenase isoenzyme was detected; a finding interpreted as secondary to resuscitation maneuvers rather than indicating a small infarct (Cobb et al, 1975, 1980a,1980b,1986). In the other study of 142 victims of out-of-hospital cardiac arrest (all ischemic heart disease patients), tachycardia/ventricular fibrillation was the cause in 95%. Sixty-two of these patients (44%) had an acute myocardial infarction; 34% had an ischemic event so called "enzymatic ischemia" and/or ST and T changes or left bundle branch block, and 22% a primary arrhythmic event (12 with, and 19 without, ST and T changes; Goldstein et al, 1981).

Another type of clinical observation deals with people, mainly ischemic heart disease patients, who die suddenly while wearing a Holter recorder. Recently, 157 cases of unforeseen sudden death or "ambulatory sudden death" occurring in such patients with stable health, and reported in literature were reviewed (Bayés de Luna et al, 1989, 1990b); cases with an acute myocardial infarction or unstable angina or in a terminal stage were excluded. Most (83%) died from ventricular tachyarrhythmia/ventricular fibrillation, a minority (16%) from brady-arrhythmia/asystole. There was no relation to exercise since sudden demise occurred mainly at rest or when a patient was sleeping. Three mechanisms of tachyarrhythmia/ventricular fibrillation were identified: (1) ventricular fibrillation preceded by only one premature ventricular contraction or by a very short run of ventricular tachycardia (8%); (2) ventricular tachycardia (more rarely ventricular flutter) that pre-cipitated into sudden death usually through ventricular fibrillation, rarely directly or through idioventricular rhythm (62%) and (3) torsades de pointes (13%). The incidence of ST changes, mainly ST depression ≥ 1 mm, in patients with ventricular fibrillation, or ventricular tachycardia leading to ventricular fibrillation, was low (13%). In contrast, cardiac pain was present in 33%, dyspnea 26% and the overall incidence of "ischemic" events higher than 70%. These observations are limited to a seriously ill population and the Holter monitor records only one or two leads. The electrocardiographic morphology of sudden death in the general population is still unknown (Bayés de Luna et al, 1990b) as is the structural counterpart of different types of cardiac arrest.

Theoretically and in accordance with the different functional forms of myocardial damage defined above, the heart may stop in a relaxed phase, in hypercontraction or after progressive failure of function. The first condition probably corresponds to asystole, associated with ischemia/anoxia, with elongation of sarcomeres. Regional hypercontraction, likely linked with intramyocardial sympathetic activity (malignant arrhythmias) has its extreme pattern in the "stone" heart (Baroldi et al, 1974). Both types of cardiac arrest whether asystole or ventricular fibrillation could occur in progressive functional failure, i.e., dilated insufficiency.

In our experience, malignant arrhythmias or ventricular fibrilla-tion never developed in the dog with intravenous infusion during one hour of increasing doses of isoproterenol or norepinephrine (Todd et al, 1985b). This may indicate that electrical instability is more likely due to a regional, altered intramyocardial release and/or reuptake of catecholamines at nerve endings rather than to blood borne catecholamines. An assumption apparently confirmed by the rarity of sudden death in patients with pheochromocytoma. However, the mechanism by which the myocardium loses its syncytial function is still a matter of speculation. Ventricular fibrillation has been defined as: "chaotic, random, asynchronous electrical activity of the ventricles due to repetitive re-entrant excitation and/or rapid focal discharge. Factors that enhance electrical synchrony facilitate, while factors that decrease electrical asynchrony hinder, the development of fibrillation" (Zipes, 1975). The major difficulty is relating electrophysiological theories, e.g., re-entry, abnormal automaticity, etc., to an anatomical substrate which is, in general, related to a myocardial infarct, or early ischemic changes often erroneously defined as contraction band necrosis. An "ischemic anisoinotropism" as asynchronous contractile status, i.e., one contracted myocell amongst normally relaxed myocells, has been proposed as a "dys-akinetic center" able to determine "micro-reentry" (Rossi et al, 1990).

Morphological identification of the type of cardiac arrest could be relevant if we are to understand the mechanism of death, especially if sudden and unexpected. In reality, anatomical substrates for the pathognomic electrocardiographic morphology of sudden cardiac arrest in general and ventricular fibrillation in particular, are still unknown. The latter is an obvious expression of an uncoordinated contractility leading to a rapid loss of pump function. In its early phase myocardial blood flow increases in the epicardium. Subsequently there is progressive flow reduction (Hottenrott et al, 1974). The heart nourishes itself so the chaotic, ineffective contraction starts a vicious circle with diminution of pump ejection inducing less myocardial nutrient flow (ischemia/hypoxia) which in turn reduces contractility. However, it is not clear what "uncoordination" means in term of the involved myocardial elements. Does it simultaneously involve all myocells or bundles of cardiac muscles or different cardiac muscles? Is there any histomorphologic equivalent of this sudden electrical storm? Any histological attempt to answer the question needs to discriminate pathological contractile status from changes due to rigor mortis. In the myocardium the latter starts 1 hour after death, resolves within 12-24 hours and may be absent in diseased hearts (Staemmler, 1961). However, little is known about how this phenomenon behaves. Again, is this postmortem contraction simultaneous in all myocardial fibers, or does it start in different cardiac muscles or bundles or cells?

In an experimental condition, normal hearts excised from anesthetized animals, using myocardial sampling at different time-intervals, it was shown that myocell contraction but not hypercontraction with marked Z line thickening, starts at 40 minutes and rapidly extends and progresses thereafter (Vanderver et al, 1981) from the subendocardium (Lowe et al, 1983). Rigor mortis, sometime named using the ambiguous and misleading term "ischemic contracture," is obviously paralleled by autolytic processes. Early separation of intercellular junctions and widening of intercellular space at disc level were occasionally seen.

MYOCARDIAL MORPHOLOGY
IN VENTRICULAR FIBRILLATION

In the ancient literature postmortem *fragmentatio* or fragmentation and *segmentatio* or segmentation of myocardial cells were mentioned. Rupture of the myocell between the intercalated discs (fragmentation) or at the intercalated disc (segmentation), is generally considered a nonvital artifact due to a microtome (Batsakis, 1968). However, fiber segmentation shows an unexplained relationship to severe contraction of the myocells (Hamperl, 1929). On the other hand, prominence of intercalated discs occurs prior to rupture of myocardial fibers in experimental extreme dilatation of heart chambers (Saphir et al, 1924; Saphir, 1933). Finally, segmentation was interpreted as an agonal event, possibly related to ventricular fibrillation (Stamer, 1907 quoted by Staemmler, 1961).

In most sudden and unexpected deaths associated with coronary atherosclerosis or in other noncoronary conditions, e.g., subjects with a positive serologic test but without manifest Chagas heart disease or patients dying following brain hemorrhage or other cardiac diseases studied in our institutions (all without resuscitation attempts), the following histologic changes were observed (Fig. 20):

1. Bundles of hypercontracted myocells with thickened Z lines contiguous to bundles of hyperdistended myocells.
2. Widening of "stretched" intercalated discs between hypercontracted fibers, often associated with segmentation.
3. Single or groups of hypercontracted myocells joined at their extremities with hyperdistended myocells. The latter may show partial or total granular disruption or fragmentation.

Any one of these "ventricular fibrillation changes" may have a different extension and topographical distribution, from focal lesions in only one region, to an involvement of the whole myocardium. They were never seen in more than 200 consecutive hearts excised at surgery for cardiac transplantation from patients with dilated cardiomyopathy, ischemic or valvular diseases or hypertrophic cardiomyopathy. This negative finding speaks against a technical artifact related to sampling and histologic procedures. Furthermore, to exclude that these changes may be secondary to ventricular fibrillation per se, we studied the hearts of 10 anesthetized, open chest dogs in which ventricular fibrillation induced, by electrical epicardial stimulus or intracoronary infusion of KCl, was maintained for 30 minutes. In no heart, were there similar "ventricular fibrillation changes" (unpublished data). Nor were they described in an experiment in calves with circulatory support by ventricular bypass pump and in which ventricular fibrillation lasted from 1-40 hours (Ghidoni et al, 1969). On the other hand, they seem different from those seen in rigor mortis.

In our opinion, their relationship to ventricular fibrillation should be settled (Vassable, 1985). Segmentation and fragmentation could be artifacts produced at the site of structures already damaged in vivo. If they express the disarray of electrical instability they may offer some indications how ventricular fibrillation works. People successfully defibrillated may have only minor, local changes, associated with rapid cardiac arrest or ventricular fibrillation following one premature beat or short run of tachycardia with minor morphologic changes; while unsuccessful resuscitation with protracted malignant arrhythmia could coincide with diffuse *myocardial damage inducing ventricular fibrillation*. We have not yet confirmed such changes.

SILENT ISCHEMIC HEART DISEASE

A patient who has clinical signs considered typical of myocardial ischemia without or with minor, nonspecific, subjective symptoms associated with a normal lifestyle is said to have *silent ischemic heart disease* (Cohn, 1989). However, a distinction must be made between people who, despite evidence of some morphologic changes typical of ischemic heart disease, e.g., coronary atherosclerosis even if severe, do not have any clinical sign and those who are without subjective symptoms and have a normal lifestyle yet have evidence of regional asynergy, ECG ischemia, etc.

Nevertheless, cases of sudden and unexpected death, (a) in apparently normal subjects, (b) without a clinical history of ischemic heart disease, (c) without evidence of ischemic symptoms, e.g., chest pain before the individual's sudden demise and (d) with histologically demonstrated myocardial infarction older than 8-12 hours, provide a unique, objective demonstration that a myocardial infarct can be *silent*. In 35 of our 208 SD subjects there were infarcts chronologically from 12 hours to less than 30 days old. When these 35 cases were compared with 200 clinically documented, fatal acute infarcts and the other 173 SD subjects without demonstrable infarction (Table 44) no significant divergencies were discovered in respect of the main morphologic variables. A higher, but not significant, frequency (14.2%) of silent infarct versus clinical infarct (2.5%) was observed in younger (<40 years) people.

In conclusion, this chapter dealt with the morphological part of the ischemic heart disease story. We synthesized the core of what a pathologist knows or believes of the natural history of the disease and of its main morphologic components. For sure, parts of this story are still defective and must be completed before ischemic heart disease is fully understood. The same can be said for the clinical side of the story; from cardiac pain and dyspnea to regional asynergy, acute or

Table 44. Silent myocardial infarct (SD people) versus clinical infarct and SD without histologic infarct

Morphologic variables	Silent infarct 35 cases	Clinical infarct 200 cases	SD no infarct 173 cases
Coronary stenosis			
<69	3	17	48
≥70	32	183	125
≥70 in			
1	12	77	41
2	12	71	48
3 or more vessels	8	35	36
Occlusive thrombus			
acute	11	83	21
old	2	30	12
Acute infarct			
size (%)			
<20	20	97	–
≥20	8	103	–
age (days)			
<2	19	70	–
2-10	4	74	–
11-30	12	56	–
Location			
subendocardial	6	26	–
internal half	18	52	–
transmural	11	122	–
Myocardial fibrosis			
absent/microfocal	31	145	148
extensive	4	55	25
Heart weight			
<500 g	23	96	98
≥500	12	104	75

chronic ischemia, electrocardiographic, echocardiographic and angiographic imagings, etc. All findings must be correlated with their pathological background, particularly when we think of structures related to coronary arteries and the myocardium that have been largely ignored, e.g., nerves or lymphatics, and to functional correlations between heart and other organs, e.g., brain and lungs.

CHAPTER 4

FUNCTIONAL SIGNIFICANCE OF STRUCTURAL CHANGES IN SUDDEN DEATH AND ISCHEMIC HEART DISEASE

After a long period of aggressive cardiology in this "catheter" era, it is time to review formulated hypotheses on the pathogenesis of ischemic heart disease. Three considerations are pertinent when the functional significance of structural parameters are reconsidered. First, clinicians and pathologists examine only what has been selected for them by already advanced disease. Second, there is difficulty distinguishing primary from secondary events in the course of the disease. Third, is the impossibility of monitoring ischemic heart disease phenomena before they happen and when they begin or end; nor do we have an experimental model of this disease. Each of these points is important when one considers cause/effect relationships in a still incomplete natural history.

In our opinion, *ischemic heart disease phenomena* are not only a hemodynamic problem but include many other factors. The aim of this chapter is to review the interrelation of variables recognized in its history, attempting to discriminate fact from fiction. We will proceed step by step, with the same sequence we did in our studies, having in mind Wilson's observation (1952): "If one doubts the necessity of controls reflect on the statement: it has been conclusively demonstrated by hundreds of experiments that the beating of tom-toms will restore the sun after an eclipse."

COLLATERALS

In coronary cineangiography, diagnostic criteria of ischemia are based on the percentage of lumen reduction found in the coronary system. Consequently, all effort is oriented to perfecting the evaluation of stenosis and relieving it. Allowing for technical pitfalls and real difficulties in obtaining correct measurements, the effect on coronary flow of a lumen reduction depends on many variables. For example, it is directly proportional to the fourth power of the radius of the lumen and is inversely proportional to fluid viscosity and the length of the tube. In particular, the pressure difference across a constricted segment is determined by pressure on the upstream side, the resistance to flow through the constricted segment and the peripheral resistance of the arteries and vascular bed distal to the constriction (Gregg, 1950). In artificial systems a maximal increase in peripheral resistance may greatly reduce flow, even in the presence of a normal lumen. In animals, prediction of flow reduction in relation to the degree of stenosis becomes more difficult because of the response of the peripheral vascular bed. In the coronary bed peripheral resistance is relatively high and generally sizable reductions in lumen are required before inflow diminishes (Gregg, 1950). Flow reduction, therefore, is difficult to evaluate particularly if we include such other variables as vessel tone and collateral flow. At present, the prevailing concept is that coronary arteries are, physiologically speaking, end arteries and even if demonstrated anatomically, collaterals cannot protect the myocardium from an acute ischemic event. In this viewpoint, nutrient flow to distal myocardium totally depends upon the amount of blood that passes the stenosed lumen of an extramural coronary artery. The rational is that even a pin-point coronary artery residual lumen (90% and 99% lumen reduction of a vessel with a diameter of 4 mm corresponds to a residual lumen of 400 μm or 40 μm respectively) allows a satisfactory flow put in jeopardy only by (a) its occlusion, leading to myocardial infarction or (b) increased metabolic demand, causing angina pectoris. Overall, this proposal is difficult to accept: too many still think of coronary arteries as rigid pipes.

In fact, the proposal was challenged when we saw the first tridimensional view of highly enlarged collateral vessels satellite to a stenosis (Baroldi, 1976, 1978, 1981). The total caliber of these collaterals exceeded by great measure the caliber of the residual stenosed lumen. We realized that an atherosclerotic stenosing plaque is not a static element but the site of integrated dynamic and biomolecular events that must be studied. As far as collaterals are concerned they are part of the normal vascular system of the human heart. Too numerous to be neglected, they are present at birth, within the whole thickness of the cardiac wall and in any cardiac region. Furthermore, extracardiac collaterals connect the coronary with adjacent arterial systems. One must remember that our findings demonstrate that in man collaterals connecting subepicardial coronary arterial branches are exceptional; the inter-homocoronary collateral system is mainly intramural.

A basic question is whether blood flow redistribution through collaterals may, or may not, prevent ischemia in the vascular territory of a stenosed or occluded coronary artery. From postmortem findings one comments that an increased collateral size can, per se, be a sign of an increased function (Baroldi, 1971). The successful compensatory mechanism can be deduced by the following observations:

1. Old total coronary occlusions are found in "healthy" subjects who died from accident yet had no ischemic heart disease clinically, nor any myocardial fibrosis.

2. Patients die from noncardiac diseases, without any cardiac disorder and/or extensive myocardial fibrosis despite occlusion or many severe coronary artery stenoses. Of 217 consecutive coronary atherosclerotic patients 46 had mild and 171 severe lumen reduction of at least one main coronary artery. An infarct was documented in only 10% and 40% respectively (Baroldi et al, 1967). In particular, a high frequency of old severe stenoses (≥90% lumen diameter) were observed without histologic evidence of a myocardial infarction or extensive myocardial fibrosis (Table 45).

3. Cases of syphilitic aortitis with bilateral coronary ostial occlusion yet without evidence of ischemic heart disease.

4. New total coronary occlusions on angiographic restudy in ischemic heart disease yet the patients do not develop a myocardial infarction (Ambrose et al, 1988).

5. The cases of marathon runners cited above (see chapter 2). In each of these conditions one might conclude that compensatory collateral function was adequate. Furthermore, in ischemic heart disease, collaterals enlarge in relation to coronary stenoses. Consequently, another fact must be considered.

6. Apparently healthy people, at their first symptoms of ischemic heart disease, generally show chronic coronary damage marked by one or more critical stenoses or occlusions which had preexisted for months or years. Again, one should state that: (a) at least until the first symptoms, the collateral compensatory function was adequate allowing a normal, if stressful, life and (b) in the natural history of ischemic heart disease its clinical onset generally occurs in the presence of enlarged collaterals because of pre existing severe atherosclerotic lumen reduction. Therefore, in most acute coronary syndrome patients, we are dealing not with normal anastomotic channels but with highly enlarged and functioning ones. However, the possibility exists that even normal collaterals may assume an immediate compensatory flow redistribution. An assumption proven in normal subjects who undergo surgical ligation of a lacerated coronary artery following a chest wound yet do not develop a myocardial infarction (Pagenstecher, 1901; Bradbury, 1942; Zerbini, 1943; Bean, 1944; Carleton et al, 1954; Parmley et al, 1958).

Other facts which support at least a partial compensatory flow redistribution are:

7. A lack of relationship between the number of occlusions and/or severe stenoses in the whole coronary arterial system and the size of an acute or old myocardial infarct. Theoretically, an increased number of critical obstructions should produce a greater degree of ischemia and a larger infarct.

8. No correlation between infarct size and the extent of the vascular territory of an occluded artery. In about half the fatal acute infarcts we studied less than 10% of left ventricular mass was infarcted This corresponds to a relative small part of the vascular territory of an infarct-related artery, which is usually occluded in the first part of its course. Most of the dependent myocardium does not undergo ischemic necrosis. On the other hand, in patients with acute myocardial infarction, hypokinesis extends beyond the occluded artery and into adjacent myocardium with adequate perfusion (Ahrens et al, 1993). A fact supported by postmortem findings in large infarcts.

All of the previous points invite one to reconsider the role of coronary collaterals in ischemic heart disease and the limitation of angiographic studies done in vivo. The latter: (a) are mainly applied to patients selected by disease; (b) cannot visualize the complexity of the intramural system, including anastomoses and (c) are restricted to a selective injection of one coronary artery. This means that few enlarged intercoronary collaterals are demonstrated while others (homocoronary, extracardiac, intercoronary from the "third" coronary artery present in about half of the human hearts) are not, because of competing nonradiopaque blood flow coming from other arteries. Furthermore, angiography in vivo shares the same criticism made of postmortem

Table 45. Old coronary (sub) occlusion (≥90% lumen-diameter reduction) without extensive (≥10% left ventricular mass) myocardial fibrosis (EF)

Source	No Cases	≥90% stenosis (%)	1	in 2	3 vess.
AMI	200	89 (100)	68 (100)	16 (100)	5 (100)
no EF	145	54 (61)	45 (66)	6 (37)	3 (60)
SD	208	75 (100)	51 (100)	22 (100)	2 (100)
no EF	133	27 (36)	19 (37)	7 (32)	1 (50)
NCA	100	40 (100)	27 (100)	11 (100)	2 (100)
no EF	81	31 (77)	21 (78)	9 (82)	1 (50)
AD	97	6 (100)	3 (100)	2 (100)	1 (100)
no EF	92	6 (100)	3 (100)	2 (100)	1 (100)

angiography; the overlapping of injected vessels does not permit correct discrimination between collateral and parent vessels. On the other hand, an appearance in vivo of a retrograde, more or less delayed filling via intercoronary collaterals of an obstructed main vessel may not indicate real nutrient flow redistribution. The main vessel distal to an obstruction may become an almost excluded channel, the blood flow having different and bypassing routes. In other words, the absence of delayed retrograde filling and/or reduced blood pressure distal to a critical stenosis may not be an incontrovertible sign of an "absent or poor" collateral flow. Equally, an absent or poor collateral flow may be an effect of extravascular compression of intramural vessels, including collaterals by irreversibly hyperdistended or hypercontracted myocardium and not the cause of regional asynergy ("hibernating myocardium").

If we assume, as seems justified, that angiographic imaging pertains to greatly enlarged collaterals only, the parameter "presence or absence or poor collaterals" reported in clinical angiographic studies may have little meaning and is of little, if any, significance. Thus, the higher degree (68%) of myocardial fibrosis of transmural biopsies at coronary bypass surgery in the absence of collaterals, versus good collaterals (29%; Schwarz et al, 1982), becomes questionable. However, some clinical angiographic findings support postmortem ones. Both, in fact, show that the largest collaterals are related to multivessel critical stenoses or to a previous myocardial infarct. Similarly, a lack of correlation between the type/extension of myocardial damage in pathologic studies corresponds to a lack of correlation between hemodynamics, number and extension of asynergic segments, metabolic factors and the presence/absence of cineangiographic collaterals (Helfant et al, 1970; Bodenheimer et al, 1977; Cohn et al, 1980; Vanovershelde et al, 1993).

We have described the secondary disappearance of intramural vessels, (including collaterals) in the infarct necrotic zone. This disappearance is proportional to infarct size; a factor rarely considered and difficult, if not impossible, to quantify in clinical angiographic studies. Furthermore, we documented in the infarcted region an increasing size of surviving collaterals (likely visible by cineangiography and postmortem angiography; Spain, 1968), findings in part confirmed by experiment (Reimer et al, 1979) and by the following clinical studies. Recanalization of a coronary artery in AMI patients using intracoronary thrombolysis is significantly less frequent (28%) in the presence of a goodly number of collaterals (distal injection of the occluded infarct-related coronary artery) than in their absence or with poor collateral numbers (55%) (Araie et al, 1990). In another clinical study, the 33% frequency of collaterals in AMI patients (intracoronary thrombolysis with complete occlusion of the infarct-related artery; 11% with subtotal occlusion) increased to 90% at the end-point, 10-14 days from onset of symptoms in patients with persistent coronary occlusion. In contrast, there was a decrease in collaterals from 38% to 7% in patients with sustained reperfusion (Rentrop et al, 1989). In a previous study in AMI patients who had persistent angiographic occlusion, 52% had no evidence of collaterals when studied within 6 hours, while almost all patients studied later (1-45 days) presented collaterals (Schwartz et al, 1984). The "disappearance" of collaterals in patients with sustained reperfusion may only indicate a new flow redistribution following the reopening of a main vessel.

Imaging in vivo is a rapidly evolving technology. Future advances in correlative understanding between functional and structural aspects can be expected. Nevertheless, we have previously listed the apparent benefits related to the cineangiographic demonstration of collaterals, i.e., prevention of postinfarct aneurysm formation, reduction of infarct size, improved ventricular function obtained in several studies (Rigo et al, 1979, etc.). We also recall the high persistence of myocardial viability within an infarct when there is collateral flow (Sabia et al, 1992b), the increase of retrograde collateral filling in about 90 seconds after sudden occlusion of a critical stenosis by an angioplastic balloon inflation (Rentrop et al, 1988); and the progressive adaptation to myocardial ischemia (*myocardial ischemia preconditioning*) by recruitment of collaterals after repetitive coronary occlusion at the site of a stenosis by angioplastic inflation (Deutsch et al, 1990; Cribier et al, 1992). The latter observations indicate that acute mechanical occlusion of a critical stenosis by balloon inflation produces a transient arrest of retrograde collateral flow which is restored in very short time. Since, experimentally, the increased size of collaterals occurs within a few days of inducing a critical stenosis (Khouri et al, 1968), one can assume that enlarged collaterals preexist angioplastic occlusion. For some unknown reason, possibly spasm of the parent vessels following this highly traumatic invasive technique, they disappear immediately after coronary balloon occlusion but return to adequate function with a normal ECG and disappearance of chest pain very rapidly. A similar preconditioning is documented experimentally in the absence of a preexisting significant stenosis. In chronic, instrumented dogs, an increase of collateral size, both demonstrated in vivo and by postmortem angiography and function, as shown by flow indices, were obtained by repetitive coronary occlusions for 2 minutes every 30 minutes continuously, night and day for 2-9 days. This structural and functional increase in collaterals prevented or reduced regional myocardial asynergy and reactive hyperemia, which reflects the degree of myocardial ischemia, secondary to transient occlusions lasting 5-120 seconds, in the absence of a chronic critical stenosis (Yamamoto et al, 1984).

Finally, the vascularization of a plaque as a possible "satellite" collateral system is apparently neglected. However, this angiohyperplasia forms a local satellite network which bypasses a stenosis by joining secondary arterial branches, proximal and distal to it and/or by connections between adventitial arteries and the residual lumen via intimal plexuses as shown by plastic casts and postmortem injection of radiopaque material (Fig. 14).

By cineangiography, even in the presence of extremely severe or subocclusive stenosis, the radiopaque menstruum immediately fills a vessel distal to a stenosis. Since the coronary injection is selective, the only route bypassing the stenosis is this *plaque satellite anastomotic* network. We do not know the compensatory role of the latter. However, one may speculate that: (a) it may contribute to flow redistribution any time there are favorable pressure gradients; (b) changes in the amount and direction of flow can be expected in relation to any new obstruction in the system; (c) reversal of flow may occur any time an increased peripheral resistance ensues caused by spasm or intramyocardial extravascular compression. Angioplasty inflation may suddenly occlude this satellite route, thus explaining acute ischemia in some cases.

In ischemic heart disease bilateral coronary ostial occlusion by atherosclerotic plaque is an uncommon finding. This pathology was not observed in our material. Nevertheless, comment on a possible role of extracardiac coronary anastomoses, particularly from bronchial arteries (Moberg, 1968) is opportune. Such anastomoses appear to be a unique source of blood supply in the presence of occlusion or severe stenosis of all coronary ostia. Indirect evidence for the compensatory function of these connecting channels is given by cases with coronary ostia occlusions due to aortitis. We had opportunity to review 11 cases from the files of the Armed Forces Institute of Pathology, Washington DC. Of these five men and six women with an age from 10-63 years and a heart weight ranging from 200-720 g, only one died suddenly, two had microfocal subendocardial necrosis and four microfocal fibrosis. Not one had a history of ischemic heart disease.

A further comment relates to collateral function in the experimental model of acute occlusion of a *normal* coronary artery. In our experience studying plastic casts from canine coronary arteries, the most frequently used animal for physio-pathological studies of the coronary circulation in relation with myocardial function, we could demonstrate extramural inter-homocoronary anastomoses connecting epicardial branches at the time of injection. In contrast, in the pig, because of very strong and persisting postmortem contraction (rigor mortis) we were unable to satisfactorily inject either intramural vessels or collaterals.

Extramural or epicardial collaterals may explain a rapid redistribution of compensatory flow after sudden ischemia in the dependent myocardial region when a normal coronary artery is acutely occluded in the dog. In fact, these anastomoses are not subjected either to extravascular systolic compression by the contracting myocardium or to its stretching (flaccid paralysis plus bulging) immediately after coronary

occlusion. This anatomical and functional condition explains why, after 1 hour of permanent occlusion which is the time needed for all
ischemic myocells to die, the infarct affects a small part of the territory supplied by the occluded artery. For instance, in dogs the circumflex branch of the left coronary artery is always the dominant artery and gives origin to the posterior descending branch. When ligated,
the resultant infarct involves only the posterior papillary muscle and
the posterolateral subendocardial layer of myocardium (Jennings, 1969).
In that animal collaterals seem to have an important compensatory
role with rapid recovery from induced ischemia in most of the dependent myocardium.

A last point to consider is recanalization of an occlusive thrombus. This has been considered an important source of distal flow redistribution (Snow et al, 1955). The subsequent occlusion by thrombi
of the new channels is interpreted as a possible cause of death (Friedman,
1967). We believe that the occlusion of such channels formed in an
occlusive organized thrombus in an area of stenosis already bypassed
by collaterals, has little significance. For example, what is the direction of flow through them, to distal lumen or adventitial vessels? Furthermore, the process of recanalization may be longer than it takes for
collaterals to develop. It is possible that such channels provide a compensatory flow function when a new critical stenosis develops in the
parent vessel of preexisting and functioning collaterals.

A basic question in the natural history of ischemic heart disease is:

*Are collaterals totally or partially inadequate to compensate an area
of acute ischemia; or may ischemia be induced by mechanisms independent of already functioning collaterals?*

CORONARY STENOSIS/OCCLUSION

CORONARY ATHEROSCLEROTIC STENOSIS

Any attempt to interpret the functional significance of coronary
atherosclerotic plaques demands knowledge of their frequency and the
degree of luminal reduction they cause *in a healthy population*. At present
a clinical approach to this problem is not feasible; any technological
type of imaging in vivo is usually applied to sick people only and not
systematically to the general population. Only a pathologist may, in
part, investigate the question by examining healthy people who die
rapidly by accident (see above and Table 4).

The morphology of an atherosclerotic plaque in an epicardial coronary
artery can be studied by histology at postmortem or by analyzing
endarterectomy or directional atherectomy specimens; or in vivo by
cineangiography. Other methods of reviewing morphology in vivo are
confined to selected patients undergoing coronary bypass surgery but
only a gross, superficial vision of a lesion is obtained by angioscopy.
Promising approaches include transesophageal and contrast echocardiography and intravascular ultrasound imaging (Lee et al, 1994).

Histology may offer structural details of the wall and intraluminal changes, particularly when serial section studies are performed. However, findings include aspects of events which occurred during the whole life of a plaque. In contrast, cineangiography offers an indirect functional imaging of the lumen and its changes seen at the time of the procedure. Despite this shadowy vision, different angiographic morphologies are described, particularly in patients with unstable angina.

Thus, a *complex* or *acute* atherosclerotic lesion/complication is correlated with the "presence of luminal irregularity or haziness with ill-defined margins, a smudged appearance, inhomogeneous opacification within the lumen or changes suggesting ulceration or plaque rupture" (Cowley et al, 1989). Using these criteria, those authors observed angiographic "evidence" of a coronary thrombus in 58% of 69 patients with unstable angina. The thrombus was occlusive in 9, all associated with well developed collaterals, and an intraluminal filling defect was found in 31. In contrast, only 5% of 20 patients with stable angina had angiographic morphology consistent with a thrombus. For complex lesions the figures were 26% and 15% respectively (Cowley et al, 1989). Similarly, in another series studied by the same criteria, intracoronary angiographic thrombus was seen in 57% of 37 patients with prolonged angina at rest. Fibrinolytic therapy improved both vascular imaging marked by reopening of narrowed segments and attenuation of ischemic symptoms. However, symptoms and signs recurred in 71% of the latter patients (Gotoh et al, 1988).

Others have classified angiographic stenoses into four categories: *concentric*, symmetric and smooth narrowing of a coronary artery; *eccentric*, asymmetric narrowing of a coronary artery subdivided in *type I* with a smooth border and a broad neck and *type II* with a convex intraluminal obstruction having a narrow base due to one or more overhanging edges or extremely irregular or scalloped borders or both and *multiple irregularities* with "three or more serial and closely spaced severe obstructions or severe diffuse irregularities in a coronary artery" (Ambrose et al, 1985a). The authors believe that a type II eccentric stenosis represents either a disrupted atherosclerotic plaque or a partially occlusive or lysed thrombus ("coronary plaque in evolution, precursor of impending infarction"). This latter type of stenosis was diagnosed in 71% of patients with unstable angina, in 16% with stable angina and in 66% of those with acute (12 hours) or recent (1-2 weeks) or healing (2-10 weeks) myocardial infarction (Ambrose et al, 1985b).

Unfortunately, coronary angiography fails to visualize all severe coronary lesions found at autopsy (Dietz et al, 1992), and angiographic findings cannot be precisely correlated with histologic ones. However, postmortem coronary angiography was compared with histology in 73 stenoses (ranging from 50% to 99% of luminal/diameter narrowing) from 39 patients dead after a myocardial infarct or following coronary bypass surgery. The angiographic stenoses were divided into *type I* (smooth borders, with hourglass configuration and no intraluminal lucencies) and *type II* (irregular borders or intraluminal lucencies). Of 35 angiographic type I stenoses only 11% presented histologically complicated plaques, i.e., those showing rupture, hemorrhage, superimposed partially occluding thrombus or recanalized thrombus, the majority being histologically uncomplicated, i.e., fatty or fibrous plaques with intact intimal surface and no superimposed thrombus. In contrast, of 38 angiographic type II stenoses, 79% were histologically complicated lesions (Levin et al, 1982). These postmortem findings indirectly support a previous report on both unstable angina and acute infarct patients (Ambrose et al, 1985). More recently it was found that angiographic "plaque rupture ("irregular lesions") is a common mechanism for progression of occlusive coronary disease but is not a mechanism whereby smooth walled plaques develop into more severe smooth walled lesions. Irregular lesions rarely become smooth lesions even after many years" (Haft et al, 1993). This proposal is difficult to accept if one considers "irregular lesions" synonymous with ruptured plaques. "The latter is not dependent on the occlusiveness of the underlying atherosclerotic plaque ... only severely occlusive (≥90%) irregular lesions commonly proceed to occlusion (50% over a mean of 2.6 years)" (Haft et al, 1993). Our experience of serial sections of atherosclerotic plaques allowed us to see in the thickened intima small arterioles with a well developed tunica media. They were connected on one side with intimal giant capillaries and on the other with a larger adventitial arterial branch. Furthermore, the latter at a different level directly communicated with the small residual lumen of the coronary artery. These vascular channels within and around the plaque may correspond to angiographic imaging erroneously interpreted as rupture or thrombosis.

A last comment requires acceptance of the concept of plaque fissuring, or rupture. We have already reported on the frequency of finding this variable in the literature. Thus, in a study with the highest frequency (89%; Davies et al, 1984) plaque fissuring was defined as "a connection between intraintimal platelet/fibrin thrombus and the lumen that is demonstrable by the presence of injection media within the plaque." One may question whether plaque rupture is an artifact due to many passages in preparing a histologic slide or whether postmortem injection per se causes fissuring. Is the source of injection material in the intima the rupture of a plaque into the lumen or does it originate from adventitial vessels connected with the hemorrhagic intima through intimal neovascularization (Fig. 13)? Greater correlation is needed if cardiologists and pathologists are to speak a common language when discussing the atherosclerotic plaque. Only then can both groups make sense of events and relate their findings to provide answers to such questions as what triggers the earliest acute event in the atherosclerotic plaque, what is its nature, and how does it interact with preexisting lesions? An estimate of all events in ischemic heart disease must include preexisting collateral flow and other acute functional factors such as spasm and regional myocardial asynergy.

Is a stenosis a cause of ischemia? Is plaque rupture the first event in acute coronary syndromes? or does a different sequence of the acute events occur?

CORONARY OCCLUSION

In general, an angiographic total occlusion has been defined as absence of forward flow of contrast medium in an involved coronary artery. The angiographic equivalent of "a thrombosis is persistent staining of intraluminal material by the radiopaque menstruum, most frequently detectable in patients with total or subtotal (>95% narrowing) occlusion" (De Wood et al, 1980); or "abrupt vessel cutoff with convex, irregular or ill-defined margins or (the) presence of contrast staining at (an) occlusion site, in association with release of occlusion or change in appearance at the occlusion site following intracoronary streptokinase or as (the) presence of intraluminal filling defects in relation to the occlusion site after patency was demonstrated" (Cowley et al, 1981, 1989). A vessel cutoff was never defined by plastic or radiopaque material injected postmortem. In all of our cases with occlusion and with or without acute myocardial infarction, the vessel distal to an occlusion was always injected via collaterals. A divergency explained by the selective injection of one coronary artery in vivo.

From the first human report of myocardial infarction (Hammer, 1878) and of experimental coronary occlusion (Cohnheim et al, 1881) more than a century ago, the role of the occlusive thrombus in ischemic heart disease has been argued. In the next paragraph we present, in summary, the pros and cons in these arguments:

ARGUMENTS IN FAVOR OR AGAINST A CAUSE-EFFECT RELATIONSHIP BETWEEN OCCLUSIVE THROMBUS AND ACUTE CORONARY SYNDROMES

PROS

1. Experimental occlusion of a *normal* coronary artery produces an infarct and/or ventricular fibrillation (sudden death).

2. Presence of an occlusive thrombus associated with the majority of large infarcts. Its location in an infarct-related artery and its "histologic" age coeval with that of the related infarct.

CONS

This model may be appropriate in some human conditions (e.g., dissecting aneurysm, embolism of a coronary artery). No experimental model exists to exactly mimic ischemic heart disease.

Not one of these facts proves or disproves that a thrombus is a primary event. Often there is no relation between vascular area/infarct size and thrombus/infarct age (see above).

PROS

3. Lack (Fulton et al, 1977) or presence (Erhard et al, 1976) of radioactivity in the occlusive thrombus of patients in whom labeled fibrinogen was injected at the onset (1 hour) of a myocardial infarct.

4. Plaque rupture is the first event followed by development of an occlusive thrombosis. This event should be associated with microembolization of atheromatous material.

5. Angiographic demonstration in vivo of coronary occlusion in 87% of AMI patients and recovery of a "thrombus" in AMI patients during emergency coronary bypass surgery. Reopening of an occluded coronary artery following intracoronary fibrinolysis.

6. Microembolization of fibrin/platelet emboli associated with microfocal ischemic necrosis in patients with unstable angina who die suddenly.

CONS

A radio-negative thrombus demonstrates only that the thrombus formed before labeled fibrinogen was injected; or alternatively a radio-positive thrombus may be due to secondary diffusion of radioactive fibrinogen into a preexisting thrombus. Both findings can neither confirm nor deny whether a thrombus is a primary or secondary event.

Rarity of atheromatous emboli within the myocardium in ischemic heart disease including unstable angina patients. One embolus only in more than 500 ischemic heart disease cases, and in 16 vessels of 4 of 25 cases (Falk, 1985) and in a single vessel of 2 of 90 unstable angina patients who died suddenly within 6 hours (Davies et al, 1986). In the 2 latter studies postmortem injection was performed and could have caused embolus dislocation.

In the unique AMI case monitored angiographically (see below) "occlusion" occurred as a secondary phenomenon and was caused by stoppage of flow because of increased intramural resistance. No thrombus formation, plaque rupture or microembolization occurred.

Most of these patients had AMI. It is impossible to discriminate between emboli and thrombosis secondary to infarct necrosis. Reported myocardial necrosis (contraction band necrosis) corresponds to catecholamine cardiotoxicity rather than ischemia (see small vessel disease below).

The dynamics in an atherosclerotic plaque are complex. We may formulate hypotheses on the sequence of events and their role in the pathogenesis of acute, and other coronary syndromes. The question remains:

Is an acute occlusive thrombosis due to plaque rupture plus micro-embolization the trigger of ischemia leading to episodes of unstable angina and/or myocardial infarct or sudden death? or is this hypothesis insufficient to explain the whole spectrum of ischemic heart disease and plaque fissuring, and thrombosis are secondary, nonfunctional effects?

DIFFERENT FORMS OF MYOCARDIAL NECROSIS

In explaining ischemic heart disease, the attention of clinicians and pathologists was, and is, mainly focused on coronary arteries and their morphologic and/or functional impairment, taking for granted that the myocardial damage is always ischemic in nature. However, the complexity of ischemic heart disease increases and jeopardizes that understanding when different patterns of pathology in the myocardium are recognized.

We observe three forms of functional myocardial damage (Table 2), each with its own specific morphology. There seems little possibility that one is related to another; consequently each must be caused by a distinct biochemical disorder (see above). Our reasoning is that any distinct pathologic entity must have a specific mechanism because the classification of diseases is based on this rule. A distinct pathogenetic mechanism always causes the same morpho/functional damage. Thus, infarct necrosis is apparently the result of a sudden nutrient flow reduction the cause of which is still unclear (see above); coagulative myocytolysis or Zenker necrosis is likely due to adrenergic stimulation or any other factor acting through free radical-mediated lipid peroxidation (Mak et al, 1988; Ferrari et al, 1990; Hori et al, 1991); and colliquative myocytolysis is likely linked with catecholamine depletion with reduced intracellular Ca^{++}, loss of K^+ and increased intracellular Na^+. Lysis of myofibrils results from prolonged beta-blocking therapy (Sun et al, 1967), hypokalemia (Emberson et al, 1969) and hypocalcemia (Weiss et al, 1966).

The conclusion, therefore, is that "metabolic" and "ion" theories of ischemic myocardial cell death due to "massive cytosolic calcium overload with inhibition of glycolysis and lack of provision of glycolytic ATP" (Opie, 1993) should consider these different forms of myocell death. To speak of "ischemic" contraction band necrosis or use, in a vague sense, the term "myocytolysis" again as an expression of nutrient flow reduction, is incorrect. Furthermore, the association of these different patterns of myocardial impairment forces us to add other pathogenic mechanisms to explain the nature of acute coronary syndromes and, in particular, its cause and complications.

If one considers the different patterns of dysfunction in the myocell many questions arise. For example, *how many times in human ischemic heart disease is there flow reduction followed by asynergy or vice versa? Does asynergy, in fact, induce flow reduction?* For instance, following dipyridamole the collateral-dependent nutrient flow greatly increases in myocardial segments with normal kinesis while it is minimal in asynergic collateral-dependent ones (Vanoverschelde et al, 1993; McFalls et al, 1993). Keep in mind that asynergy may be due to all three types of myocardial damage. Again, *what is the meaning of blood flow measurement without any knowledge of contractile status and their chronological relationship?* And finally, *should we consider "ischemic necrosis" any morphologic form found in the myocardium or distinguish these different forms, including nonischemic ones, to understand pathogenic mechanisms, complications and mode of death?*

LESIONS OF INTRAMYOCARDIAL OR INTRAMURAL CORONARY ARTERIAL VESSELS (SMALL VESSEL DISEASE)

The concept that platelet aggregation has a role in myocardial ischemia derived from experimental intracoronary and intraventricular infusions of adenosine diphosphate (Jorgensen et al, 1967, 1970). The latter produced transient circulatory collapse, ECG ischemic changes, eventual ventricular fibrillation and a transient fall in circulating platelets due to aggregation in microcirculatory vessels and myocardial "infarct." Animals made thrombocytopenic or with platelets refractory to ADP did not show evidence of severe circulatory changes or myocardial necrosis. The conclusion was that ischemic heart disease may be caused by microcirculatory platelet aggregation secondary to ADP released from different sources, e.g., tissue injuries, lysis of red blood cells, etc., (Mustard et al, 1969) and particularly from erythrocytes damaged when crossing a stenosed atherosclerotic plaque (Brain et al, 1962), platelet adhesion being inhibited by adenosine (Born et al, 1964).

The only morphologic lesions found in human intramural arterial vessels that might possibly cause an acute coronary syndrome are aggregates of platelets and/or fibrin/platelet thrombi or emboli (Fig. 21). Already defined above such findings are reported often in ambiguous terms and without a clearcut distinction whether they formed in situ or embolized from proximal sources. Few postmortem studies on sudden death (Table 35) demonstrate these lesions; several angiographic reports on AMI ischemic heart disease patients with normal coronary arteriography take for granted that this pathogenic mechanism exists. However, in fatal infarct cases with minimal or no lumen reduction of the coronary arteries there was no evidence of primary intramural lesions (Eliot et al, 1974).

A recent review emphasizes the complexity of platelet/endothelial interactions and the seeming ability of some diseases, such as atherosclerosis, diabetes mellitus, hypertension, uremia, hypercholesterolemia and preeclampsia, to impair release of endothelium-derived relaxing factor and nitric oxide (vasodilatation) and antiaggregatory platelet factors (anticoagulation and fibrinolysis) from one site and to promote the endothelial release of vasocontrictive substances and platelet aggregating factors from other sites (Ware, 1993). Experimental coronary constriction of 60-80% in the dog determines a cyclic blood flow reduction secondary to transient obstruction of the stenosed vessel. It is not clear if this transient obstruction is due to platelet aggregation or spasm (Folts et al, 1982) or both.

The last intramural change worth mentioning is medial hyperplasia obliterans (Fig. 22). Found in papillary muscles and columnae corneae in both controls and ischemic patients, it can be observed in endomyocardial biopsy and erroneously interpreted as a cause of ischemia.

Is it justified to continue to hypothesize that small vessel diseases is a pathogenic mechanism in ischemic heart disease/sudden death even including in this term all possible morphologic forms of intramural vascular impairment proposed in literature?

FINDINGS IN SUDDEN
AND UNEXPECTED CORONARY DEATH

In the previous chapter, the significance of pathology in the subgroup of *sudden coronary, expected death* in ischemic heart disease patients with known unstable angina was discussed. Here, the morphologic findings in another pattern of acute coronary syndrome, namely *sudden and unexpected coronary death* are reviewed.

In general, and apart from specific acute damage, e.g., coronary thrombus, infarct or Zenker necrosis, plaque inflammation, heart rupture, most cardiac sudden deaths show old lesions (Tables 31 to 40), including arterial dysplasia in the conduction system and atherosclerotic plaques, when they are considered only in terms of causing lumen reduction. The question then is, how does an old lesion explain an acute event such as sudden death? For example, we refer to the sudden and unexpected death of a young girl at the end of a swimming race: she had an enormous fibroma of the left ventricle (Heath 1969). Also, the two cases of marathon runners described above, one dead suddenly and unexpectedly and the other expectedly, both with critical old coronary artery stenoses and severe myocardial scar. Such hearts with old, severe and extremely extensive coronary lesions yet capable of performing in stressful physical or mental conditions is not an uncommon finding. This invites modification of the old expression a "heart too good to die" because of the absence of significant lesions (Beck et al, 1960) into a "heart too bad to live" emphasizing the enormous functional capability of this organ and its ability to compensate even in the presence of extensive damage. One notes that in forensic medicine the detection of severely obstructive coronary atherosclerosis, per se, is often thought sufficient to permit a diagnosis of sudden coronary death. However, the same degree of severe vascular lesions are often found in healthy people dying by accident and in patients dying for noncardiac diseases (Tables 4 and 6). One may, therefore, question the correctness of this diagnosis. In other words, old lesions, including those in the conduction system, can be regarded, at best as predisposing factors in sudden death.

The question then is how an acute event such as sudden and unexpected death can be explained by morphologic findings?

CHAPTER 5

PATHOLOGIC BACKGROUND AND PATHOGENESIS OF SUDDEN DEATH/ISCHEMIC HEART DISEASE: A PERSONAL VIEWPOINT

E ach segment of chapter 4 ended with a question to prompt discussion on the relationship between structure and function in sudden death/ischemic heart disease. This section is devoted to our viewpoint derived from our data and interpretations.

CORONARY ATHEROSCLEROTIC PLAQUE GROWTH

CAN GROWTH OF THE ATHEROSCLEROTIC PLAQUE EXPLAIN ISCHEMIC HEART DISEASE?

Recently the genesis, evolution and role of a coronary atherosclerotic plaque in ischemic heart disease was brought up-to-date in the following manner:

"The initiation of atherosclerosis may result from blood flow oscillatory shear stress in certain vascular sites (bending points, bifurcations, etc.) producing chronic minimal injury resulting in functional alteration of the arterial endothelium (type I injury): experimentally, this is potentiated by atherogenic risk factors such as hypercholesterolemia, hypertension, immunocomplexes, viral infections and tobacco smoke. Such minimal injury leads to the accumulation of lipid and monocytes (macrophages) and subsequently, toxic products released by the macrophages produce damage of the intimal surface with denuding endothelium (type II injury or damage) which attracts platelets; all of these cells release growth factors, prompting migration and proliferation of smooth muscle cells and producing a "fibro-intimal lesion" or the outside of the capsule of a predominant "lipid lesion." The lipid lesions surrounded by a thin capsule tend to be small and rupture easily, causing type III injury or damage; that is, they are soft and weak, contain large numbers of macrophages, which may release collagenase and elastase to form abscesses, and by their location, are under the effect of flow shear forces. After plaque disruption there is thrombus formation: when thrombi are small, they can become organized and contribute to the growth of the atherosclerotic plaque; when thrombi are large and occlusive, they lead to the acute coronary syndromes. New data suggest that, at the time of plaque disruption, certain "thrombogenic" risk factors modulate the degree of thrombogenicity and, thereby, the growth of the plaque versus the various acute coronary syndromes. Aside from the need for better understanding of the basic biology of atherogenesis, emphasis on identifying and modifying the primary atherogenic and thrombogenic risk factors should continue for primary prevention. Also, new approaches should focus on the identification, stabilization, and regression of the small "lipid plaques" prone to rupture (these are not necessarily angiographically apparent) as well as on the use of better and safer antithrombotic agents for prevention of progression" (Fuster et al, 1992).

This quotation has the merit of synthesizing the current viewpoint on the cause and pathogenic mechanisms of acute coronary syndromes. Our impression, however, is that this model is biased by experimental data obtained in animals fed cholesterol diets (Ross, 1993). A model which may correspond to arterial lesions found in human familial or acquired hypercholesterolemia but not to those observed in the general population with or without ischemic heart disease. In the latter, the absence of platelet aggregates or platelet/fibrin thrombi, subendothelial lipoprotein/macrophage, monocyte infiltration (foam cells), fissuring in 1519 coronary sections with normal lumen and in 1315 coronary sections with mild (≤69%) luminal stenosis and minor (<600μm) intimal thickness supports the existence of two types of atherosclerotic plaque each with a different natural history: they are the *hypercholesterol plaque* and the *smooth myocell hyperplastic plaque*. We have already described a possible progression of the atherosclerotic process in the latter. Keep in mind that the nature (? monoclonal;Benditt, 1974) and stimulus of the first intimal changes, i.e., nodular smooth muscle cell hyperplasia and sequelae are still not explained just as there is no demonstration of rupture and thrombosis of *small* lipid plaques. The concept of *different types of plaque growth* suggests that regression may be different in each type of plaque; a hypercholesterol plaque being more prone to stop or regress if hypercholesterolemia is normalized.

CORONARY STENOSIS AND ISCHEMIA

Is a Critical Luminal Stenosis the Cause of Ischemia?

The association of coronary atherosclerosis and ischemic heart disease is well documented. However, more accurate proof is needed to confirm the current opinion that a critical luminal stenosis causes ischemia. The frequency and degree of atherosclerotic coronary damage is significantly higher in acute coronary syndromes, i.e., acute infarct and sudden/unexpected death, which occur in chronic ischemic heart disease patients versus "1st episode" patients (Table 6). However, in the latter 11% of acute infarct and 35% of sudden/unexpected death patients had a normal lumen or a noncritical (≤69%) stenosis in the whole coronary arterial system. On the other hand, noncardiac patients showed figures similar to the mean values found in sudden/unexpected death cases. Even 39% of healthy people dying by accident had one or more critical stenosis. Apparently there is no direct relationship between a critical stenosis and ischemic heart disease. A fact confirmed by the absence of relationship between the degree and extension of critical atherosclerotic damage and subsequent clinical course and between infarct size and the number of critical stenoses (Table 22).

When we speak of myocardial ischemia the latter is interpreted as an acute phenomenon capable of explaining acute coronary syndromes. However, regional hibernation of the myocardium has been interpreted as a consequence of *chronic ischemia* due to old obstructions in the coronary arterial system. Therefore, a chronic flow reduction which temporarily stops myocardial cell function only, without damaging myocell structure (viable myocardium) is a captivating hypothesis. Nevertheless, the idea of chronic coronary ischemia contrasts with all data which support the concept of an adequate compensatory function of collaterals (see next paragraph).

COLLATERAL FUNCTION

Are Collaterals Totally or Partially Inadequate to Compensate for Ischemia?

The narrowing of a coronary artery lumen by atherosclerotic plaque raises a question of the role of collaterals in preventing ischemic heart disease. We have listed all facts from which an adequate compensatory collateral flow can be deduced. At the same time, we indicate how inadequate angiographic imaging is in visualizing the collateral system; "good" angiographic collaterals being secondary to an infarct without any functional meaning.

Amongst facts supporting an adequate compensatory flow redistribution by collaterals (see above) in acute ischemic syndromes are two that are very important: (a) the first ischemic episode generally occurs in the presence of one or more chronic and critical stenoses in one or more of the main epicardial arteries (see below for mild angiographic stenosis in acute coronary syndromes). This indicates that up to his or her first ischemic symptom or sign, a man or woman was able to handle a normal, often stressful life despite preexisting severe coronary atherosclerosis. The only explanation is that the latter is compensated by collaterals as confirmed by (b) an experimental critical stenosis in the dog maintained for 5-7 days producing a dramatic increase in collateral size capable of protecting the animal's heart from subsequent occlusion of the residual lumen (no infarct or dysfunction or malignant arrhythmias; Khouri et al, 1968). One might conclude that an acute ischemic syndrome starts independently of, and despite, an adequate collateral flow.

PLAQUE RUPTURE

DOES RUPTURE OF AN ATHEROSCLEROTIC PLAQUE TRIGGER AN ACUTE CORONARY SYNDROME?

There is some evidence that in unstable angina and acute myocardial infarction a plaque can be the site of dynamic events that can be related to the acute pattern of disease. However, at autopsy no differences were shown in different categories of patients with mild/moderate or severe stable angina at effort and relieved by rest or nitroglycerin, or with unstable angina mainly at rest and often prolonged in respect to the severity of coronary atherosclerosis (Guthrie et al, 1975). The major difficulty is recognizing all dynamic factors linked with the acute coronary syndrome. Fissuring or rupture of a plaque and secondary thrombus, with or without embolization and their supposed angiographic equivalents (type II eccentric stenosis, or luminal lucencies, filling defects, etc.) are only a few of the variables seen in an active plaque. In plastic casts of atherosclerotic coronary arteries, which have the advantage of a tridimensional image, different patterns of "irregular" lumen and recanalized channels can be seen. From such a study and from serial sections of plaques it is obvious that a plaque, particularly when located in an infarct-related artery, is the site of different, concurrent dynamic factors. At present we can only speculate about their sequence when looking at an *active plaque*, since we do not have an experimental model to reproduce the events nor can we follow it in humans. Any attempt to define plaque "activity" must consider all anatomical and dynamic factors recognized to this point. They include:

1. Luminal stenosis of any degree.
2. Satellite collaterals (homo- and intercoronary anastomoses), the anastomotic network around the plaque (connections between adventitial arterioles-capillary network, intimal vessels and residual main coronary lumen; (Baroldi et al, 1967; Zamir et al, 1985) and the recanalized channels of an even-

tual organized thrombus.

3. Spasm of the coronary artery and the status of the tunica media.
4. Inflammatory reaction in the plaque, particularly its relation to the regional nervous system.
5. Vascularization/hemorrhage in the plaque.
6. Role of endothelial, smooth muscle, macrophage and mast cells in releasing growth factors or thrombogenic and/or vasoactive substances.
7. Regional myocardial asynergy with increased intramural resistance (extravascular compression) and flow blockage in a related main subepicardial artery (increased wall stresses).

Recently, emphasis has been given (Entman et al, 1993; Buja et al, 1994) to a marked "inflammatory" process mainly represented by macrophages, described in atherectomy material from patients with unstable angina or non-Q-wave myocardial infarction (Moreno et al, 1994) as well as at the immediate site of a ruptured or eroded plaque with thrombosis in patients dying from acute myocardial infarction (Wal et al, 1994). In defining the inflammatory lymphocytic and plasma cell infiltrates in atherosclerotic plaques of ischemic heart disease patients, we distinguished between primary inflammatory processes and secondary macrophage reaction to tissue injury. It is not surprising that patients with active, dynamic plaques have recurrent tissue injuries linked with many other functional factors and associated with a macrophage reaction. The latter does not necessarily have a cause/effect relationship with the acute coronary syndrome.

At present, the claim that plaque fissuring is the starting point of an acute coronary syndrome is unproven and apparently contradicted by iatrogenic plaque rupture following angioplasty (see below) and by the rarity of atheromatous emboli and coronary artery dissecting aneurysm. If fissuring is so common one might expect a higher frequency in ischemic heart disease. A finding not observed in our material or reported in literature.

CORONARY OCCLUSIVE THROMBOSIS

IS THE ACUTE THROMBUS DUE TO PLAQUE RUPTURE THE CAUSE OF MYOCARDIAL INFARCTION AND SUDDEN DEATH?

In our review of arguments about causal factor(s) of ischemic heart disease, we noted a need to examine a phenomenon at its onset and during its development. All previously reported clinical/angiographic and postmortem studies deal with patients examined, at best within 1 hour of the clinical onset of their acute ischemic syndrome or dying after a relatively long period, possibly with a variety of therapeutical maneuvers and drugs applied. Even 1 hour is a long period in which to distinguish primary from secondary events.

At the Italian Institute of Clinical Physiology (Pisa) it was possible to follow a particular patient and all coronary angiographic and clinical events prior to and after a myocardial infarction he suffered during coronary angiography. Twelve months later, the patient had a heart transplant because of progressive, intractable cardiac failure and the excised heart was studied (Baroldi et al, 1990). This 45 year-old man had unstable angina pectoris for 2 weeks. A diagnostic coronary angiography was performed while he was clinically stable. The procedure showed both anteroseptal and anterolateral hypokinesis with a critical stenosis in the right coronary artery and two critical stenoses of the left anterior descending branch (LAD), one upstream and one downstream of the origin of the second diagonal branch. Aortic pressure was 137/70 mm Hg and left ventricular pressure 130/12 mm Hg. The first ECG change (downsloped ST segment) *without any subjective symptom or other clinical and angiographic sign* was noted following the fourth LAD injection. Because of persistent ECG changes, another four LAD injections were performed *without any changes in angiographic images or any clinical or subjective modifications.* Only during the last injection did the postenotic tract of the vessel become fainter and disappear. Again, the image of *LAD occlusion was not associated with other clinical and angiographic parameters or subjective symptoms.* An intracoronary vasodilator and Ca^{++} antagonist failed to restore blood flow. Following an intracoronary bolus (50,000 U) and intracoronary infusion of urokinase (10,000 U/min) for 20 minutes, ST changes and T-waves tended to normalize with an image of recanalization. However, despite continuing urokinase infusion, the ECG changed again with LAD reocclusion. At this time, approximately 90 minutes after the first ECG ischemic changes, the patient felt mild chest discomfort. Percutaneous transluminal angioplasty was then performed successfully with reopening of both proximal and distal LAD stenoses. Nevertheless, there was no benefit to the patient who experienced increasing chest pain and marked ST-segment elevation. Repeated contrast injection into the LAD demonstrated a progressive disappearance of the vessel starting from its distal portion and extending to its origin from the left main trunk. Since another balloon attempt failed to restore flow, the patient underwent emergency aortocoronary artery bypass surgery. The entire LAD was filled by an easily aspirated coagulum. Accurate probing documented a normal lumen without appreciable narrowing at any site. The LAD and implanted graft distended as soon as the clamp was released, but, as shown by a flow-meter, had no flow. Vessel and graft remained patent at repeated probing, but flow was never restored. The patient recovered from a large antero-lateral-septal infarct and was discharged home 15 days later. However, because of progressive, intractable heart failure without other episodes of ischemic heart disease, he had a heart transplant 12 months later. The excised heart showed a massive antero-lateral-septal left ventricular scar (approximately 30-40% of left ventricular mass) with an aneurysm of the antero-lateral wall. Multiple microfoci of fibrosis were detected in remaining parts of left and right ventricles without evidence of any change in intramural vessels. The myocardium showed a diffuse loss of myofibrils (colliquative myocytolysis). The LAD and corresponding vein graft presented severe lumen reduction (LAD 90-95%, vein graft 70-80%) along their whole courses. An organized occlusive thrombus was found at the site of surgical anastomosis. The first part of the right coronary artery was occluded by an old, organized thrombus in an area 90% stenosed by atherosclerotic plaque. The left circumflex branch was mildly stenosed (50%) in its distal part. Atherosclerotic plaques in all coronary arteries revealed severe atheroma, calcification, and lymphocytic and plasma cell inflammation, histologically.

As far we know, this is the only case in the literature where it was possible to follow clinical events before and after a myocardial infarction and to have pathological documentation without superimposed agonal or resuscitative effects. The case demonstrates the following points:

1. The first ischemic ECG change occurred and persisted for 20 minutes, without angiographic evidence of coronary occlusion, chest pain or angiographic alteration of the LAD stenoses.

2. At 20 minutes angiographic occlusion was documented without chest pain or worsening of ECG changes or other clinical parameters. Only 70 minutes after coronary angiographic occlusion and 90 minutes from the first ECG change did both the ECG worsen and chest pain occur, despite successful angioplasty.

3. A rapid sequence of up-to-date therapeutic interventions failed to restore permanent coronary flow. Only brief, temporary periods of reflow were documented during intracoronary urokinase (reocclusion despite continuous infusion of the drug) and after successful angioplasty. Paradoxically, ECG and chest pain worsened following the latter procedure.

4. The disappearance of the LAD started from its distal portion and progressed retrogradely to its origin from the left main trunk.

5. Evidence at surgery of a patent LAD filled by an easily removed coagulum.

6. Pathologic documentation of a large infarct in the territory of LAD, corresponding to the hypokinetic zone diagnosed before infarction. Absence of an infarct in the territory of the right coronary artery which was occluded by a recanalized thrombus at a site of a severe stenosis. Absence of any changes such as old fibrin/platelet and/or atheromatous emboli in intramural vessels.

All facts indicate that in this case of unstable angina, the acute syndrome (infarction) started without documented angiographic occlusion of a coronary artery with the latter demonstrated only 20 minutes after the first ECG changes. Therefore, the occlusion appeared to be secondary (no evidence of spasm) and, per se, did not promote any new objective and subjective signs for approximately 70 minutes. It seems unlikely that the acute ischemic syndrome started at angiographic occlusion. Furthermore, the nature of the angiographic occlusion was documented by inspection at surgery and overall by its retrograde progression from the distal part of the vessel to its origin and not to the site of stenosis where the left circumflex branch had unrestricted flow. All data indicate that this angiographic occlusion was a *pseudo-occlusion* due to flow blockage by intramural resistance with blood coagulation, not thrombosis, in the infarct-related LAD. There was no evidence of any type of intramural embolization, while "no reflow phenomenon" (Summers et al, 1971; Majno et al, 1967; Kloner et al, 1974; Gavin, 1983) seemed unlikely due to the short and rare periods of reperfusion and absence of malignant arrhythmias.

One may only speculate on the possibility of spasm in intramural arterial vessels (no increased blood flow noted after intracoronary vasodilator), or extravascular compression by dysfunctioning myocardium marked by worsening of the preexisting hypokinetic zone with increased myocardial stretching by intraventricular pressure. However, questions arise. They include: (a) how many angiographic occlusions in general and in particular how many of the 87% of acute infarct cases with total angiographic occlusion observed within 4 hours (De Wood et al, 1980) had the same type of "pseudo-occlusion" seen in this case; (b) how many "layered thrombi" of platelets, fibrin and red cells recovered at surgery (De Wood et al, 1980) seen in atherectomy material (Escaned et al, 1993; Rosenschein et al, 1994) or by intravascular ultrasound imaging (Lee et al, 1994) or that were suspected in angiographic imagings are only coagulated blood? Note that in this patient a large transmural infarct was fully established in a relative short time (20-70 minutes), despite instant and appropriate therapy; chest pain being an unreliable signal in timing the event.

According to postmortem studies not all coronary occlusions are pseudocclusions (Roberts et al, 1972; Buja et al, 1981). We know that in acute infarcts, mainly at the level of an atherosclerotic plaque with critical stenosis we have, in about 50% of fatal AMI, an occlusive thrombus. Its frequency is related to infarct size and, in our experience, is minimal (20%) in infarcts less than 10% of left ventricular mass and maximal (86%) in ones greater than 50% of left ventricular mass. This divergence may explain discordant reports in the literature, including angiographic and pathologic mismatch (see below). However, the frequency of a thrombus is only one variable which may have very little significance when we have to establish its functional meaning and its cause/effect relationship with an infarct and/or sudden death. In our studies, beside findings related to infarct size, the presence of an occlusive thrombus correlated with a severe (≥70%) degree of lumen reduction, the concentric shape of a plaque, its length, an atheromatous type of plaque and its lymphocytic and plasma cell inflammatory reaction. In other words, the variable "thrombus" is a multivariant phenomenon. If one selects only very large infarct cases with luminal narrowing of the related artery of more than 90% and a concentric, long, atheromatous and inflamed plaque the probability of finding an occlusive thrombus is 100%. This, however, does not prove that the thrombus caused the infarct. On the contrary, when one considers all dynamic aspects of a plaque, the hypothesis of secondary thrombus formation seems justified. A critically narrowed atherosclerotic plaque means that a functioning collateral system formed by satellite, homocoronary and/or intercoronary anastomoses and by a network of communicating channels around and within the plaque bypasses the stenosed lumen (Fig. 24). This flow redistribution, with reduced anterograde flow counterbalanced by retrograde collateral flow distal to the stenosis, implies its hindrance within the tortuous residual lumen. Angiographically, to (during systole) -and-fro (during diastole) flow can be seen. This hemodynamic background may act, per se, with stasis of blood around and within the greatly vascularized plaque, or may be associated with: (a) a mechanical action of the contracting myocardium on the coronary wall especially in exertion (Black et al, 1965); (b) coronary spasm and (c) extravascular compression of nonfunctioning myocardium with increased peripheral resistance and further blockage of flow in the related artery both in the residual lumen and in connected intimal/adventitial vessels. All factors which may explain the sequence of events in a dynamic or active plaque causing fissuring or rupture, hemorrhage (vasoactive or thrombogenic substances) and thrombosis (Fig. 23). Bear in mind the occurrence of plaque hemorrhage mainly in the infarct-related artery; the reduced fibrinolytic activity of an atheromatous plaque and the increased coagulability any time there is tissue necrosis. In a patient who died within 5 hours of angiographically demonstrated coronary occlusion likely due to spasm, a mural thrombus at the site of a 70% stenosis without rupture of a plaque was observed in a serial section study. Clinically, the last episode was typical of an infarct but it was not demonstrated histologically because of a short survival time (Maseri et al, 1978).

The hypothesis of secondary thrombus formation is supported by the frequent occlusion of a stenosis after surgical bypass grafting (Aldridge et al, 1971; Griffith et al, 1973). In a functional sense, the bypass flow is equivalent to a satellite collateral flow. On the other hand, if one accepts the concept of thrombus formation secondary to hindrance of distal flow associated with thrombogenic and/or vasoactive substances, the progression to occlusion of an already critical stenosis by subsequent mural thrombosis is another secondary event without functional significance. In other words, clinical angiographic aggravation of a critical stenosis or stenoses already bypassed by collaterals may not necessarily worsen ischemic heart disease in an ischemic sense. This is also demonstrated experimentally (Khouri et al, 1968).

On this subject, one notes an increasing number of angiographic reports (see above) defining a thrombotic occlusion at the site of a noncritical coronary atherosclerotic stenosis in an infarct-related artery. This is in contrast to postmortem findings. Pathologists agree that where an occlusive coronary thrombus is demonstrated it forms at a site of critical luminal stenosis ($\geq$70% lumen-diameter). This association was observed in 93% of fatal myocardial infarcts with a thrombotic occlusion and in 100% of cases of sudden and unexpected death with this finding. In reviewing a series of 190 AMI patients (117 associated with reopening of an occluded coronary artery by intracoronary fibrinolysis; Cowley et al, 1981; Ganz et al, 1981; Mathey et al, 1981; Reduto et al, 1981) we found that 63 patients had an angiographic evaluation of the residual coronary artery stenosis following recanalization. The residual stenosis was critical in 84% of these patients. In contrast, in other studies comparing coronary angiographs before and up to a month after an AMI, authors found that "in the majority (66%) of subjects the myocardial infarction occurred because of the occlusion of a coronary artery that did not contain an obstructive (more than 50% diameter narrowing) stenosis on a previous coronary angiogram" (Little et al, 1988; Hackett et al, 1989). However, in these studies the first coronary angiogram was performed a long time (mean 706 $\pm$ 685 days with a range from 4-2,298 days) before infarction. Of 42 cases only 4 had coronary angiography 3 weeks before their AMI; 3 patients had "mild" coronary stenoses. Furthermore, there was no demonstrable occlusion at the time of acute infarction. In a larger series of 283 low risk, medically treated ischemic heart disease patients, 2 angiograms were performed 4.6 $\pm$ 0.1 years apart. At restudy 60 (21%) of 283 patients had developed a total of 75 new coronary artery occlusions and only 19% of them had a clinically recognized infarct. The majority (85%) of infarct-related coronary artery lesions were not hemodynamically significant (0-75% stenosis) at initial study (Webster et al, 1990). Nevertheless the angiographer's viewpoint is: "In many patients (78%) who subsequently developed myocardial infarction, prior angiography revealed lesions that were <50% occlusive in the infarct-related artery. Although the degree of narrowing in these arteries just before the onset of infarction was unknown, it was assumed that a more significant narrowing in the infarct-related artery had not slowly developed before the acute event. We suspect that this may have occurred because progression of coronary artery disease at restudy was uncommon in noninfarct-related lesions. Therefore, disruption of a mild or moderate atherosclerotic plaque with resultant thrombosis and total or subtotal occlusion probably explained the myocardial infarction. In patients with a previously normal appearing infarct artery, we assume that some degree of diffuse coronary disease was indeed present, but was not detectable by these angiographic techniques" (Ambrose et al, 1988). In the same study a second group of 15 patients had 18 new total occlusion mainly (61%) at the site of previous critical (>70%) stenoses.

The assumption that occlusive thrombi develop at the site of noncritical stenoses seems weak for many reasons. First, it has never been demonstrated at autopsy. Second the very high frequency of noncritical plaques even in healthy controls (Table 4) speaks against small plaques being prone to rupture and developing associated occlusive thrombi. Third, the previously mentioned angiographic studies were, in general, performed months or years before the infarct. Without knowledge of the "angiographic" degree of stenosis at the time of the latter, one can only defer to postmortem observations (Table 13). Furthermore, the concept of a persistent mild stenosis in an infarct-related artery suggested by a lack of progression of stenoses in noninfarct-related vessels does not consider the effects on plaque progression caused by regional-related asynergy. In the quoted case report from the Pisa Institute, after 12 months the left anterior descending branch and its vein graft, normal at surgery, showed severe lumen reduction due to atherosclerosis along their whole course. This raises the possibility that progression of atherosclerosis is related to dysfunction of dependent myocardium. Blockage of intramural flow may enhance all conditions, i.e., physical, functional, neurogenic and biochemical from several cellular sources which stimulate progression: the latter being much slower in vessels related to normally functioning myocardium. As previously mentioned, another possibility is that the inflammatory reaction in the plaque may increase progression particularly in a radial, stenosing direction. In our acute infarct cases the infarct-related *active* plaque was significantly shorter and severely narrowed.

Finally, one notes that an infarct may occur in the absence of a previous mild or severe stenosis (Eliot et al, 1974) and pseudo-occlusion or blood clotting because of increased intramural resistance. This may explain "incomplete lysis of thrombus" in mild/moderate stenoses found in acute infarct patients undergoing intracoronary fibrinolytic therapy (Brown et al, 1986). On this subject, the frequent failure or inadequacy of acute recanalization following intracoronary fibrinolysis (about 50% according to Brown et al, 1986 and 39% in the study of Vogt et al, 1993) may be due to the type of occlusion; pseudo-occlusion with easy lysis of a coagulum, whether spontaneously or by fibrinolytic agents, compared to true occlusion by a thrombus with less satisfactory lysis. Thrombi are present at autopsy in about 50% of the total population of fatal acute infarcts. We note that thrombolysis after acute myocardial infarction, in contrast to experimental temporary coronary occlusion, does not affect the prevalence of complex ventricular arrhythmias (Turitto et al, 1990).

MYOCARDIAL DAMAGE

CAN DIFFERENT FORMS OF MYOCARDIAL DAMAGE EXPLAIN DIFFERENT CLINICAL PATTERNS OF ISCHEMIC HEART DISEASE?

In the past 20 years innumerable human and experimental studies were instituted to reduce infarct size. The rationale is that a smaller infarct has a more benign course and that around an acute infarct is an ischemic border zone, prone to infarction. It must receive rapid therapeutic protection. We show that more than 50% of acute fatal infarcts are small, the size being independent of the degree of coronary damage. Furthermore, survival was shorter in small infarcts. Therefore, the first conclusion is that a malignant clinical course is not necessarily related to infarct size. Second, in all AMI cases we were unable to document an extension of the original infarct, i.e., a central area of infarct necrosis of whatever age surrounded by more recent infarct necrosis. Similarly, we were unable to identify lesions described experimentally after temporary coronary occlusion, the so-called wave front phenomenon in reflow necrosis. It must be stressed that our cases were selected, avoiding as much as possible, iatrogenic effects, invasive techniques or resuscitation maneuvers. On the contrary, the finding of Zenker necrosis at the periphery of an infarct and in the noninfarcted myocardium suggests that rather than an ischemic border zone we may speak of normal myocardium at risk of catecholamine or catecholamine-like myotoxicity (Baroldi, 1975,1984). Arrhythmogenic complications and/or death are likely related to the degree and maintenance of the latter; positive technetium-99 stannous pyrophosphate myocardial scintigrams correlated with complicated postinfarct course and "myocytolytic degeneration" (Buja et al, 1977).

We know that blood flow is increased around an infarct (Hood, 1970), confirmed by the polymorphonuclear infiltration starting at its periphery. Also increased contractility (Goldstein et al, 1972) is likely stimulated via mechanoreceptors (Malliani et al, 1979) consequent to the loss of contraction of infarcted myocardium. In experimental infarction both Zenker necrosis and ventricular fibrillation were prevented by beta-blockers (Baroldi et al, 1977) as was myocardial necrosis after transient ischemia (Sommers et al, 1972) or following denervation in permanent coronary occlusion (Jones et al, 1978), Lidocaine (Nasser et al, 1980); superoxide dismutase (Przyklenk et al, 1986) or regional preconditioning (Przyklenk et al, 1993). Abnormal myocardial function was also prevented by beta blocking agents (Tomoike et al, 1978). In comparison, in sudden and unexpected coronary death in the absence of an infarct, a similar cardiotoxicity linked with malignant arrhythmias may be due to adrenergic stimulation by other, still undetermined causes such as inflammation of pericoronary nerves adjacent to the media, and/or spasm, regional asynergy, etc. One point needs further investigation. Acute and severe flow reduction, no matter whether caused by coronary spasm or extravascular compression of intramural vessel by stretched or hypercontracted myocardium, etc., may rapidly stimulate via nervous reflexes the intracardiac adrenergic system, the "electrical" cause of death perhaps being linked more with the latter than with the former and mortality reduction obtained in some countries being mainly due to beta-blocker therapy.

In chronic patients, a third main cause of complication and death is heart failure. Colliquative myocytolysis is a sign of this condition. It must be explained whether the failure is due to a loss of contractile proteins or to a still unknown metabolic disorder leading to a primary deficit of contraction with subsequent loss of myofibrils.

Serum enzymes do not discriminate between different types of myonecrosis. Furthermore, in our opinion, in acute infarcts they are washed from the peripheral Zenker necrosis zone, where flow is maintained or increased, rather than from infarct necrosis which quite rapidly becomes a sequestered, avascular area. The relationship between high levels of serum enzymes and a malignant course may be due to severe adrenergic cardiotoxicity.

A last practical note concerns the avascular area interpreted dynamically. It is mainly due to stretching of infarcted myocardium (intraventricular pressure) already histologically documented within 15 and 30 minutes respectively in rat (Hort, 1968) and dog (Baroldi et al, 1977) after coronary occlusion. The postmortem lack of injection likely corresponds to a diminished intramural flow in the dead tissue in vivo. This implies failure of any therapeutic vascularization within a short time of an infarct's onset (see reported AMI case).

SMALL VESSEL DISEASE

IS THERE ANY MORPHOLOGIC PROOF THAT SMALL VESSEL DISEASE CAN CAUSE ACUTE AND CHRONIC CORONARY SYNDROMES?

Total coronary vascular resistance resides in vessels with a diameter larger than 100 μm and its regulation is extremely complex. It is controlled by several factors including autoregulation, O_2 consumption, sympathetic stimulation, serotonin, vasopressin, adenosin, endothelin, etc. (Marcus et al, 1990).

Although James (1967) considered small vessel disease a factor in ischemic heart disease and Saffitz et al, (1983) reported one case of sudden death with amyloidosis of small coronary arteries, we found no particular morphologic lesion of intramural vessels to explain acute coronary syndromes. In the literature, obliterative intimal thickening is described in arteries of the conduction system ("fibromuscular dysplasia") and linked to sudden death. This change is also observed in healthy controls and there is no proof that it induces acute coronary syndromes, i.e., sudden death (see below).

In terms of obstructive small vessel disease the main debate relates to platelet aggregates. In discussing their role in sudden death/ischemic heart disease two aspects must be distinguished. One concerns their aggregation and fibrin/platelet thrombi formed in situ, the other pertains to platelet or fibrin/platelet masses embolized from thrombosed proximal vessels.

Platelet adhesiveness can be determined by several factors, including catecholamines (Bridges et al, 1966) not necessarily linked with an atherosclerotic plaque; for example, endothelial derived factors are important. The question is whether an obstruction caused by platelet aggregates or the release of vasoactive amines by them with resultant local vascular spasm could explain ischemic episodes and trigger sudden death. When reported (Table 35) the number of vessels occluded by platelet aggregates in cases of AMI is small. In our observations there was no difference in this finding between SD cases and controls. Thus the relationship is problematic and deserves further study. On the other hand, in human pathology some conditions exist which can be defined as experiments of nature. Thrombotic thrombocytopenic purpura is one. This is a unique disease marked by a diffuse occlusive microangiopathy of intramural arterioles plus diffuse platelet aggregation in normal arterioles. Furthermore, it is characterized by other anoxic factors such as severe hemolytic anemia plus ADP, hemorrhages or neurologic disorders, including convulsions with increased cardiac activity. No one of the 39 TTP cases we studied had symptoms or signs of ischemic heart disease or died suddenly and unexpectedly. In 31% microfoci of Zenker necrosis were observed. Similarly, in 53 cases of sickle cell anemia, the plugging of small vessels by sickled erythrocytes (documented in vivo; Knisely, 1961) was never associated with myocardial damage of any type (Fig. 48). One also notes a normal left ventricular performance and an absence of ECG changes or MB isoenzymes of creatine phosphokinase during sickle cell crisis (Val-Mejias et al, 1974).

The other aspect is embolization of platelet or fibrin/platelet masses from an occlusive or mural thrombus in the main artery supplying an ischemic area. This finding seems peculiar to patients with unstable angina who die suddenly (and "expectedly") within 6 to 24 hours. In 80% of these patients an infarct has been documented histologically (Table 35). It is difficult to discriminate how many such vascular lesions are emboli rather than fibrin/platelet thrombi formed locally in intramural vessels within infarcted myocardium as a secondary phenomenon. They are never seen outside the infarcted myocardium in man and in experiments. A progressive blockage of flow (avascular area) by the stretched, necrotic myocardium plus local factors such as neutrophils, wall degeneration, etc., could explain secondary thrombosis in situ. Furthermore, such emboli have been described in AMI patients treated with coronary thrombolysis (Waller, 1991), and one may ask if other therapeutic procedures, e.g., resuscitation attempts, etc. induce embolization. Terminal therapy was not reported in most pertinent studies. One can not exclude spontaneous platelet emboli from a related ruptured plaque of a coronary artery. The question is whether these emboli are the cause of microinfarcts leading to sudden death. The number of occluded vessels is not reported or when reported is astonishingly low. For instance, amongst 260 sections from zones perfused by a thrombosed artery only 72 microemboli were found in 29 sections (Falk, 1985). A finding which raises doubts about a claimed cause/effect relationship. More important, is that the associated myocardial necrosis, called a "microinfarct" in the literature, has clear-cut histological features of microfocal often confluent Zenker necrosis. We have stressed that this lesion is not ischemic and cannot be defined as infarct necrosis. Rather, adrenergic overstimulation causes it. One notes that platelet aggregation has never been demonstrated in the early phases following experimental infusion of catecholamines either by electron microscopy (Todd et al, 1985a) or by Cr-labeled platelets (Moschos et al, 1978).

Practically, in the natural history of ischemic heart disease and related sudden death other types of small vessel diseases do not exist. Platelet aggregation or embolization, even in a subset of patients with unstable angina, seems an unlikely, ischemic factor, particularly if one consider that 38% of unstable angina patients are hypersensitive to spasmogenic stimuli in respect of acute infarction (20%) and stable angina (4%) (Bertrand et al, 1982). Spasm could induce plaque rupture plus embolizing thrombus. Moreover, no beneficial clinical effects occurred in several studies using thrombolytic treatment in unstable angina (Neri Serneri et al, 1992). The hypothesis of ischemic plugging by, and/or vasoactive substance released from, polymorphonuclear leukocytes (Mazzone et al, 1993; Entman et al, 1993) has no basis in pathologic findings. In the natural history of ischemic heart disease neutrophils appear 6-8 hours after onset of an infarct, when this lesion is fully established. It is unlikely that these leukocytes aggravate the lesion. Neutrophils are not part of atherosclerotic plaque inflammation, are only seen in infarct necrosis and are rare in reflow necrosis; a finding not observed in human acute coronary syndromes. Experimental infarct size reduction by abolishing neutrophil cytotoxicity (Amsterdam et al, 1993) needs further investigation.

A final comment relates to distal embolization of atherosclerotic plaque material and/or thrombus formation during balloon angioplasty (Saber et al, 1993). The major mechanism of dilatation by this procedure is plaque fracture (Waller, 1991). This should imply microembolization of pultaceous or eventual thrombotic material as well as thrombus formation. In two autopsied cases, thrombotic material was observed in a few intramural vessels (Waller, 1991). In experimental angioplasty in normal swine producing eccentric medial disruption and the formation of a crater, thrombus was totally absent (Gravanis et al, 1993). The latter was also absent in human plaques fractured by angioplasty (Wanibuchi et al, 1992). Furthermore, successfully dilated coronary lesions with an angiographically visible dissection are no more likely to develop restenosis and are not associated with a worse clinical outcome at 6-month follow-up than are dilated lesions without visible dissection (Hermans et al, 1992).

One notes that sudden death or myocardial infarction is a rare event following balloon angioplasty (4-5% acute complications). This indicates that embolization following plaque rupture may have little, if any, functional significance. On the other hand, the rarity of atheroemboli in sudden death/ischemic heart disease cases without emergency and invasive procedures, including postmortem injection of radiopaque material, suggests that spontaneous plaque fracture in coronary arteries is a rare event and secondary to other mechanisms such as spasm or stasis related to increased peripheral resistance. These mechanisms may prevent embolization.

A COMPARISON OF SUDDEN CORONARY DEATH VS MYOCARDIAL INFARCT VS UNSTABLE ANGINA

A comparison of findings in *unexpected* versus *expected SD* cases reveals the same acute lesions, divergencies being more quantitative than qualitative. When sudden and unexpected death is compared with selected cases of acute fatal infarction the major differences are: (a) a higher distribution of critical atherosclerotic stenosis in AMI *1st episode* versus SD *1st episode* (Table 6); (b) a reduced frequency of occlusive thrombi in SD *1st* (8%) versus SD *2nd episode* (28%) and overall versus AMI (42%) without variation in AMI *1st and 2nd episode* (Table 12); (c) absence of any type of intramural arterial thrombi but fibrin/platelet ones secondary to histologically demonstrable infarct necrosis; (d) a lower frequency (3% in noncritical and 20% in critical stenosis) of intimal hemorrhage in atherosclerotic plaques (Table 7b) in respect of AMI (16 and 43% respectively); (e) a minor (but not significant) frequency and extension of inflammatory plaque reaction in SD than in AMI cases and (f) the presence of catecholamine necrosis in all acute coronary syndromes.

From these data one notes that cardiac arrest in ischemic heart disease and sudden death is mostly due to malignant arrhythmias resulting in ventricular fibrillation, particularly in the early phase of infarct necrosis and independent of its size. Sudden death, however, is not synonymous with an infarct since the majority of people resuscitated by defibrillation and most who die suddenly while monitored by a Holter device do not show the ECG pattern of an acute "Q-wave" infarction. Therefore, in sudden coronary death, we should distinguish the following two possibilities: first a malignant fatal arrhythmia associated with focal Zenker necrosis that appears before an acute myocardial infarct becomes obvious histologically. Second, an intramyocardial, regional sympathetic storm may occur within a patient not developing a myocardial infarction. Coagulative myocytolysis, and possibly *ventricular fibrillation damage* as previously described, is the morphologic sign of this storm. The hypothesis is apparently supported by:

1. The Cardiac Arrhythmia Suppression Trial (CAST) which was prematurely terminated because of a high mortality in patients not receiving beta-adrenergic blocking agents (Peters et al, 1994);

2. Reduction of sudden death in patients with ischemic heart disease by lipophilic betablockers, which easily pass the blood-brain barrier and increase cardiac vagal tone and electrical stability of the heart (Wikstrand et al, 1992);

3. Clinical demonstration of sympathetic overactivity, i.e., significant relation between number of ischemic episodes or the overall duration of silent ischemia and norepinephrine spillover both at rest and after cold test, in active unstable angina in respect of inactive unstable angina, stable effort angina and controls (Schwartz et al, 1992; Neri Serneri et al, 1993; McCance et al, 1993);

4. By a higher frequency of sudden death in patients with a heart rate ≥ 65 beats per minute indicating low parasympathetic activity vs. ≤ 65 beats without relation with other risk factors (Algra et al, 1993) and

5. Experimental reduction of ventricular fibrillation threshold by betablockers (Baroldi et al, 1977; Anderson et al, 1983) likely related to calcium influx (Clusin et al, 1982).

The adrenergic system, fully developed in mammals, is an adaptation system which allows rapid adjustment in heart rate, contractility, airways, peripheral resistance, venous tone, glycogenolysis, platelet adhesiveness, coagulability, etc. Therefore, this is an alarm system which permits an animal to react quickly and effectively to acute situations either by aggression, escape or other emergency reactions (Cannon, 1942; Raab, 1970; Kubler, 1992, 1994). In ischemic heart disease the sympathetic system may go out of control and aggravate myocardial damage by inducing progressive cell injury and ventricular tachyarrhythmias. Myocardial ischemia is a unique situation of increased sympathetic stimulation with increasing neurotransmitter release, diminished activation and regulation of receptors and temporary activation of effect or enzyme leading to extension of infarct size and the induction of threatening ventricular arrhythmias (Kubler, 1992, 1994). We emphasize that rather than "extension of infarct size" we should speak of "adrenergic cardiotoxicity," coagulative myocytolysis being the morphologic hallmark of an out-of-control sympathetic response. The question is whether in any case of sudden death in which this morphologic hallmark is obvious ("mural" coronary artery; Morales et al, 1980, isolated congenital coronary artery anomalies; Taylor et al, 1992b, right ventricular arrhythmogenic dysplasia; Thiene et al, 1988), we may speak of a similar sympathetic storm, no matter what its cause.

In this context, sudden death cases without "critical" coronary atherosclerosis must be mentioned. In our experience, amongst 28 cases (all SD 1st episode) with a normal coronary lumen or a lumen reduction less than 50%, the frequency of Zenker necrosis was 78%. This suggests that a sympathetic storm may occur in the absence of severe coronary atherosclerosis. In turn, it emphasizes a need to study the whole sudden death population without selecting only cases with severe coronary damage and second, the inappropriateness, in forensic medicine practice, of linking sudden coronary death to severe coronary atherosclerotic obstructions alone. Furthermore, sudden death linked with malignant arrhythmias in any coronary condition, e.g., congestive heart failure in chronic coronary ischemia (Lesch et al, 1984); in animals with sequential intracoronary embolization, (Sabbah et al, 1992) or in noncoronary conditions, e.g., familial hypertrophic cardiomyopathy (Anderson et al, 1983; Hecht et al, 1993), myxomatous mitral valve (Pasternac et al, 1982; Chesler et al, 1983), systemic amyloidosis, (Falk et al, 1984), congestive heart failure (Packer, 1985; Parmley, 1987), cardiomyopathies (Brandenburg, 1985; Goodwin et al, 1976, 1978, Maron et al, 1978; Marcus et al, 1982; Oparil et al, 1985; Hecht et al, 1993), radiation-induced coronary obstruction (Angelini et al 1985) or systemic sclerosis (Bulkley et al, 1978) merits further investigation to establish the presence of histologic signs of catecholamine cardiotoxicity. The latter were present in sudden and unexpected death in a case of acquired immunodeficiency syndrome with lymphocytic myocarditis (Baroldi et al, 1993) and in seropositive subjects with Chagas disease without a subjective or clinical history of heart disease but with extensive myocarditis associated with ventricular fibrillation damage (unpublished data).

Recently, by scintigraphy, abnormalities were demonstrated in sympathetic innervation related to ventricular arrhythmia (denervation supersensitivity) in both ischemic heart disease (Calkins et al, 1993) and in the absence of coronary disease (Mitrani et al, 1993). Similar nerve destruction seems to be the cause of the stunned myocardium (Ciuffo et al, 1985). Following 25 minutes of coronary occlusion, there is a contractile response to norepinephrine infusion or bretilium tosilate but not to sympathetic ganglia stimulation; a fact that must be considered in the presence of regional asynergy and related to the mechanical effect on nerve endings following irreversible myocardial stretching or hypercontraction within a normal beating myocardium. One must remember that regional sympathetic reinnervation takes time and may be heterogeneous (Wilson et al, 1993) and that an experimental transmural myocardial infarction produces sympathetic denervation in noninfarcted sites, apical to the area of necrosis (Barber et al, 1983).

The heart/brain relationship (Skinner, 1985) is still a matter for investigation (Lown et al, 1977, 1979). In acute brain lesions focal Zenker necrosis is described in the heart (Connor, 1969) and prevented experimentally by a betablocker (Hunt et al, 1972). In experimental subarachnoid hemorrhage arrhythmias develop with a sudden increase in intracranial pressure. In animals with both vagi and heart sympathetic innervation sectioned but with an intact spinal cord, arrhythmias were delayed and could not be correlated with intracranial pressure. These findings suggested that arrhythmias could be produced either by direct autonomic discharges to the heart or by increased circulating and tissue cathecholamines (Estanol et al, 1977). In animals with coronary occlusion psychological stress, e.g., electrical shock in dogs with and without acute infarct, can alter ventricular threshold of cardiac vulnerability and provoke major arrhythmias (Corbalan et al, 1974).

A more precise histological documentation is needed in all cases of different behavioral type (Kahn et al, 1987) who die suddenly following emotional distress; "myofibrillar degeneration" has been observed in victims of homicidal assaults without internal injuries (Cebelin et al, 1980), particularly in ischemic heart disease patients in whom helplessness or hopelessness were basic feelings (Engel, 1971). In turn, this raises the still undetermined mechanism of sudden death in aboriginal people ("voodoo death" Cannon, 1957). Intense emotion is a common denominator of these psychological states (Lynch et al, 1977; Eliot et al, 1985) in which a loss of balance between sympathetic and parasympathetic modulation may produce tachycardia and ventricular fibrillation, bradycardia or asystole.

We note that "passive" emotion or fear, per se, seems insufficient to elicit sudden death. For instance, no epidemics of sudden death were reported during War World II, despite numerous stressful conditions in very large groups of people of different race. On the other hand, a classic pattern of clinical transmural anteroseptal myocardial infarction without infarct necrosis has been described in two patients, one with a cerebral infarct and the other with a primary brain tumor. At autopsy, only "focal myocytolysis" and severe coronary atherosclerosis were observed (Duren et al, 1976). These cases support a brain/heart relationship in man in the presence of coronary atherosclerosis, and emphasizes the lack of ECG specificity in discriminating different forms of myocardial necrosis. "Ischemic" ST depression is the ECG signs of acute Zenker necrosis following infusion of noradrenaline or isoproterenol in the absence of flow reduction (Todd et al, 1985b), and had a high frequency in patients resuscitated from out-of-hospital cardiac arrest at an exercise test (Sharma et al, 1987). Sympathetic dysfunction is regional since no arrhythmias were demonstrated experimentally by systemic intravenous infusion of catecholamines (Todd et al, 1985b). In contrast, severe malignant arrhythmias occurred in a few dogs with norepinephrine infusion in one coronary artery (unpublished data).

CAUSE AND PATHOGENESIS IN SUDDEN DEATH/ ISCHEMIC HEART DISEASE—ALTERNATE HYPOTHESES

The previously mentioned *unifying theory* of ischemic heart disease is based on mechanisms affecting atherosclerotic plaques in coronary arteries, namely plaque fissuring, thrombosis and microembolization. It is attractive both because of its simplicity (few variables) and because it prompts interventional activity in both prevention and treatment. Recently, this approach was expressed as follows: "the incidence of plaque rupture appears to be reduced in patients receiving cholesterol-lowering therapy, beta-adrenergic blocking agents and, possibly, angiotensin-converting enzyme inhibitors and antioxidants. Not all ruptured coronary plaques produce an acute coronary syndrome. The consequences of plaque rupture depend on the extent of thrombus formation over the fissured plaque. This is determined by flow characteristics within the vessel as well as the activity of the thrombotic and fibrinolytic systems. Recent advances in cardiovascular molecular biology, coronary diagnostic techniques and cardiac therapeutics have opened windows of opportunity to study and modify the factors leading to plaque rupture. The local modification of gene expression to alter plaque composition and to elucidate and subsequently inhibit the prothrombotic and fibrinolytic defects that promote coronary thrombosis may, in future, prevent plaque rupture and its consequence" (MacIsaac et al, 1993). In replying to this and another opinion that it "is hardly credible that there should be continuing debate about what is ostensibly so simple a morphologic problem: the relationship of coronary thrombosis to acute myocardial infarction" (Davies et al, 1976) one may paraphrase Hurst's sentence, "Some words prevent learning," published in 1967 into "some morphologic findings prevent learning." If the functional meaning of a morphological finding is reviewed carefully and its correct meaning resolved, we may begin to seek truth.

What may seem so simple does not reflect facts. Sudden death/ischemic heart disease appears an integrated set of phenomena of which plaque fissuring is only one morphologic finding. We present above much data that make us doubt the value of the simplistic, unifying theory and the cause/effect relationship between an occlusive coronary thrombus and all forms of myocardial necrosis. Rather, we believe that these data support a secondary role for plaque rupture, thrombosis and embolism and that metabolic mechanisms rather than ischemia explain some complications and deaths in acute and chronic ischemic syndromes. Amongst morphologic variables we note a significantly higher frequency and extent of a lymphocytic and plasma cell inflammatory response in coronary atherosclerotic plaques in patients with ischemic heart disease. These lesions, strategically located around nerves adjacent to the media allow new working hypotheses. This inflammatory reaction is different from the macrophagic response present in the intima of plaque. Thus, we provide different pathogenic mechanism:

The lymphocytic plasma cell inflammatory reaction in a plaque alone, or by inducing "irritation" or "degeneration" of medial nerves releases substances that may cause vasospasm or affect regional cardiac contractility. These changes invoke:

1. Myocardial infarction and other forms of myocardial necrosis.
2. Ventricular fibrillation without myocardial ischemia.
3. Coronary artery spasm which includes myocardial ischemia and secondary phenomena in coronary arteries (e.g., fissuring, thrombus and embolism).

The peculiar tropism for advential nerves in the adjacent media of the observed plaque inflammation begins when plaque progression reaches the proteoglycan accumulation stage, being already present in small plaques that cause no or minimal lumen reduction and are not visible by angiography. This active process progresses within a plaque and is significantly more frequent and diffuse in plaques of ischemic heart disease patients. As in any chronic, recurrent inflammatory process inactivity may alternate with activation triggered by many factors. This could explain the high ischemic heart disease variability in different patients with equal coronary damage. This process could act in either of the following ways:

Irritation		*Release of*
or		*active substance*
degeneration		*from*
of		*lymphocytes or*
adventitial nerves		*plasmacells*
	resulting in:	
Spasm	and/or	*Abnormal*
of		*regional*
coronary		*myocardial*
vessels		*contractility*

leading to
Regional hypokinesis
(nonfunctioning viable myocardium)

Any condition which adds to regional hypokinesis such as an increased intraventricular pressure because of increased contractility of the myocardium around hypokinetic zones will result in
Regional dyskinesia

with intramural extravascular compression which nullifies the nutrient flow to the myocardium. According to the duration of flow stoppage the following may develop:

Angina	or	*Reflow*	or	*Infarction*
Pectoris		*Zenker*		
less than		*necrosis*		
20 minutes		20-60 minutes		>60 minutes

In all of these conditions, an increased intramyocardial release of catecholamines, elicited via nervous reflexes around the asynergic zone, can be expected. In turn, adrenergic cardiotoxicity may result in malignant arrhythmia/ventricular fibrillation.

This theoretical line (Fig. 24) was suggested by the *avascular area phenomenon* in acute infarct necrosis and is supported by many clinical findings which include our case report, and the fact that changes in contractility precede pain and ECG alterations (Nesto et al, 1987) as shown also in ambulatory sudden death patients (Taki et al, 1987). In this, we note that even in the endstage of congestive heart failure, sudden cardiac arrest may be caused by ventricular tachycardia/fibrillation in subjects with prior myocardial infarction who underwent heart transplantation (Lum et al, 1989).

The fact that sudden death cases are defibrillated without evidence of a myocardial infarction or that sudden death occurs in ECG monitored patients without evidence of ischemia, supports a concept that ventricular fibrillation is linked to *primary regional catecholamine cardiotoxicity*. Obviously there is no way of proving or disproving this possibility because we lack an experimental model and objective documentation of contractility immediately before sudden death. Nevertheless, one can not exclude a regional adrenergic overstimulation in which several factors act or interact. Impairment of myocardial metabolism precedes ventricular fibrillation (Corday et al, 1977).

Coronary occlusive spasm results in sudden ischemia immediately followed by myocardial dyskinesia and further adrenergic overstimulation via nervous reflexes. This situation is comparable to experimental acute coronary occlusion with rapid (before an infarct can be demonstrated histologically), death due to ventricular fibrillation linked with catecholamine cardiotoxicity. Premature ventricular contractions after an acute myocardial infarct depend on the residual ventricular ejection fraction and not reperfusion (Marino et al, 1994). In a few cases (Maseri et al, 1978; Roberts et al, 1982) in whom histologic control was possible, coronary artery spasm was always associated with an atherosclerotic plaque with severe luminal stenosis; an observation confirmed by intravascular ultrasound (Yamagashi et al, 1994). Spasm is obviously related to a functioning media. Despite its reduction at a plaque site (Arbustini et al, 1991), local medial changes are still compatible with a constrictive function.

We note that spasm has not been demonstrated in normal extramural coronary arteries or intramural vessels in man. At present, the only solid evidence supporting the concept of spasm in an extramural coronary artery seems associated with atherosclerosis. Here, the role of adventitial perinerve inflammation or adventitial mast cells (Forman et al, 1986) needs further investigation. Furthermore, the variability in extension of nerve impairment may explain a lack of relationship between the size and topography of infarct necrosis (or hypokinesis) and coronary arterial lesions.

In this, we wonder about the meaning of systemic monocytic or granulocytic activation seen clinically (Neri Serneri et al, 1992; Mazzone et al, 1993) in acute coronary syndromes. This activation may be more related to myocardial damage (infarct necrosis for granulocytes, coagulative myocytolysis for monocytes) than to the inflammatory process we are discussing. The latter is a local reaction strictly related to the atherosclerotic lesion. Elevation of C-reactive protein and serum amyloid A protein in severe unstable angina may be related to it (Liuzzo et al, 1994). At present, there is no proof that spasm occurs in intramural vessels with a more or less developed tunica media such as small arteries, arterioles, metarterioles, precapillaries. One cannot exclude that microvascular spasm shown in the Syrian hamster (Factor et al, 1982) is caused by extravascular compression of asynergic myocells. Zenker necrosis is the typical acute lesion seen in these animals.

IS "ISCHEMIC" OR "CORONARY" HEART DISEASE THE CORRECT DEFINITION?

Colloquially, in defining the epidemic of coronary heart disease or acute coronary syndromes, the term "coronary" is synonymous with ischemic factors and is used to define an atherosclerotic stenosing/occlusive lesion responsible for all clinical patterns. The present review suggests a different meaning. In particular, silent or nonsilent ischemia is not a major determinant of sudden and unexpected death. The latter is frequently triggered by a ventricular premature depolarization with a preceding short-long heart cycle that likely produces dispersion of refractoriness in an arrhythmic substrate (Gomes et al, 1989). Complications and death seem more related to myocardial "toxicity" than ischemia while onset may or may not be caused by the latter. In reality and in contrast with other opinions (Ambrose, 1992), each acute syndrome presents a specific morphology and clinical pattern which makes it an entity, irrespective of whether one transforms into another. In the acute infarct syndrome the basic myocardial lesion is a consequence of abolishing nutrient flow, the cause of which is under discussion. However, complications and death are not often related to infarct necrosis and its complications, e.g., heart rupture, embolism from intraventricular thrombus, very large infarct size, etc., per se. In unstable angina different components may coexist, namely adrenergic overdrive leading to several disorders and possible temporary regional asynergy, the nature of which is still undetermined (chronic ischemia or regional nerve impairment?). Autonomic neuropathy in diabetic patients leads to an increased sympathetic tone which could explain their high frequency of sudden death (Jacoby et al, 1992). Overall in *coronary heart disease* a sympathetic disorder seems to prevail and the benefit of betablocker therapy may be related to this mechanism. Furthermore, through the link between the sympathetic nervous system and stress one may speculate that in the general population and in most coronary heart disease patients the beginning of an atherosclerotic plaque, i.e., a nodular smooth muscle cell hyperplasia is related to a sympathetic neurogenic disorder of vessel wall control likely elicited by hemodynamic stress factors particularly active in extramural coronary arteries. In other words, our data support the concept of a prevailing role for sympathetic activity in the whole natural history of coronary heart disease, particularly if one considers the multiple effects of adrenergic hypertone on the blood, arterial wall, hyperlipidemia (lipolysis), etc. (Eisenberg, 1966; Levine et al, 1964; Kaplan 1987, 1988; Yamori et al, 1987; Cruickshank et al, 1987; Ablad 1988; Wikstrand et al, 1988; Ross, 1993) and the linkage between adrenergic stimuli and immunologic response in relation to cardiovascular changes (Benshop et al 1994; Maisel 1994).

===================== CHAPTER 6 =====================

SUMMARY

The aims and concepts of this book and the sequential steps by which it was constructed, were mentioned in the preface. To critically revisit ischemic heart disease the rational was (a) to start with a detailed summary of our morphologic studies; (b) to synthesize data from the literature; (c) to outline present knowledge on the natural history of coronary heart disease by reviewing histories of any single morphologic parameters which may play a role; (d) to discuss their significance by comparing imaging in vivo and postmortem and (e) to present our interpretation of the phenomena which occur in the natural history of this disease. Such an approach implies some unavoidable repetition. The latter, however may stress crucial points and be helpful according to the Latin dictum *repetita iuvant* (repetitions help in understanding).

Our data and findings observed when specific methods and definitions are used, allow the following points:

1. Coronary plaque rupture, luminal thrombosis and both intramural emboli or fibrin/platelet thrombi can be interpreted as secondary phenomena that cannot explain acute coronary syndromes.

2. Each acute coronary syndrome is an entity with different causal and pathogenic mechanisms. The latter are still hypothetical.

3. Myocardial infarct necrosis is caused by ischemia mainly produced by extravascular compression of intramyocardial vessels secondary to stretching of hypokinetic myocardium because of increased intraventricular pressure. Hypokinesis is the first clinical sign of infarct necrosis.

4. Infarct size, when infarct necrosis only is correctly measured, is not generally related to a malignant clinical course or death, nor to the degree and number of severe coronary artery stenoses.

5. The supposition postulated by images of mild stenoses associated with plaque rupture plus occlusive thrombus is not confirmed by pathological studies.

6. A malignant clinical course and cardiac arrest are mainly due to alteration of autonomic nervous control leading to arrhythmias (ventricular fibrillation) or congestive heart failure. The fundamental mechanisms are likely caused by primary myocardial cardiotoxicity unrelated or indirectly related to ischemic hypokinesis as in cases of infarct necrosis.

7. "Catecholamine" myocardial necrosis (Zenker necrosis) is always present in any acute coronary syndrome. Instead of infarct necrosis extension, the wavefront phenomenon is mainly caused by catecholamine cardiotoxicity. No morphologic evidence of extension of infarct necrosis exists when a distinction is made between the latter and Zenker necrosis.

8. Another form of myocardial necrosis (colliquative myocytolysis) is a sign of myocardial insufficiency in the chronic coronary syndrome. The latter is characterized by extensive, substitutive myocardial fibrosis. However, two major patterns can be distinguished: one in which infarct necrosis prevails (*chronic coronary infarct syndrome*) and the other mainly due to catecholamine cardiotoxicity (*chronic catecholamine cardiomyopathy*), both leading to congestive heart failure.

9. In acute coronary syndromes the atherosclerotic plaque is the site of several events which may explain luminal and intimal changes secondary to hemodynamic or medial or nerve impairment. In our definition an *active plaque* is related to an inflammatory process which may derange regional contractility via nerve involvement, release of active substances resulting in coronary spasm or myocardial asynergy.

10. Sympathetic overtone seems the major cause of many disorders in coronary heart disease, including plaque growth, malignant arrhythmias and sudden cardiac arrest.

11. We have to distinguish between the *smooth myocell hyperplastic coronary plaque* seen in coronary heart disease and the general population, and the *hypercholesterol coronary plaque* obtained experimentally by a hypercholesterol diet or observed in familial or acquired hyperlipidemia in man.

12. In acute and chronic coronary syndromes there is no good evidence of small vessel disease of any type.

Our alternative viewpoint is an attempt to answer three main questions: (1) why we develop ischemic heart disease; (2) why we have a variable clinical course without a definite recovery and (3) why we die. The suggested mechanisms, not yet or poorly considered, may help complete the mosaic in understanding the disease. Our working hypotheses do not deny benefits obtained by angioplasty, coronary bypass surgery and/or fibrinolytic therapy. All of these invasive techniques with plaque disruption and/or denervation may determine drastic changes in plaque structure which abolish functional disorders, e.g., spasm, regional asynergy, etc. Furthermore, fibrinolytic agents, generally infused when an infarct is already well established, may help normalize secondary acute hypercoagulability, thus reestablishing blood flow with a more rapid recovery of contractility in noninfarcted myocardium and lysis of coagulated blood in an infarct-related artery as soon as blood flow returns. However, it must be remembered that streptokinase itself may improve contractile function in the ischemic left ventricle (Fung et al, 1984).

Our data and concepts are an invitation to reconsider the linkage between atherosclerosis and the current epidemic of coronary heart disease; avoiding premature and misleading theories and proposing only working hypotheses. Atherosclerosis is an old disease of human beings, being present, in Egyptians of high social class, as shown by their mummies (Ruffer, 1911). Why and how in particular socio-economic conditions it becomes the background of disease in some organs is still a matter for research. Any idea or concept based on solid facts merits further investigations to substitute preconcepts with truth.

As pathologists we make a plea for a high autopsy rate to allow continuing detailed morphologic studies of acute and chronic coronary syndromes. Without that information and a multidisciplinary approach to the problem of coronary heart disease each of us studying the condition can be likened to blind persons examining parts of an elephant. The study of man is man. Each investigator provides snippets of information that must be synthesized to achieve full understanding.

CHAPTER 7

ILLUSTRATIONS

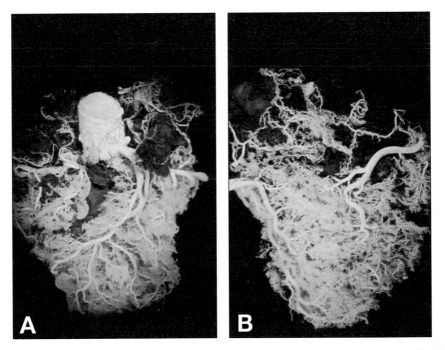

Fig. 1. Tridimensional cast of coronary arteries from a normal human heart showing both extra-and intramural vessels. (A) anterior view, which includes a cast of the proximal ascending aorta and (B) posterior view. Reprinted with permission from Baroldi G. In: Silver MD, ed. Cardiovascular Pathology, 2nd Ed. New York: Churchill Livingstone Inc.,1991a:487.

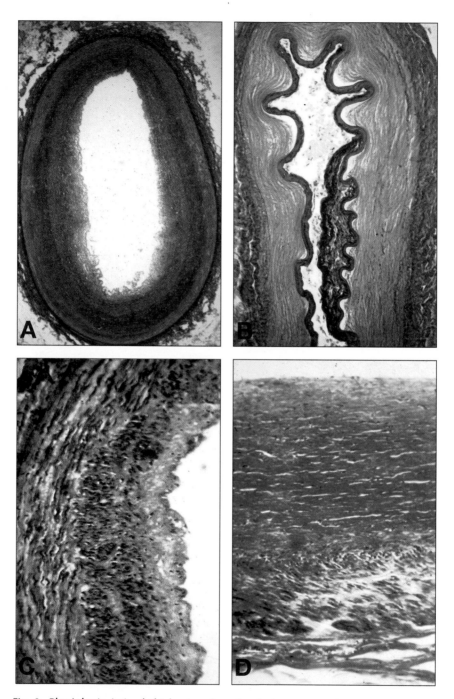

Fig. 2. Physiologic intimal thickening, found only in extramural coronary arteries. It becomes circumferential at the end of the second decade and does not alter the vessel lumen. (A) The intima is thicker than the media in this 18 year old man. (Weigert elastic X 30). (B) In noncoronary muscular arteries the finding illustrated in A is absent or minimal. Middle cerebral artery of the same subject (Weigert elastic X 60). With increasing age this intimal thickening progressively loses myocellular and elastic components becoming a fibrous intimal layer. (C) LAD in 20-year-old woman (lumen to right: Gomori X 50); (D) LAD in 85 year-old woman (lumen at top: Gomori X 100).

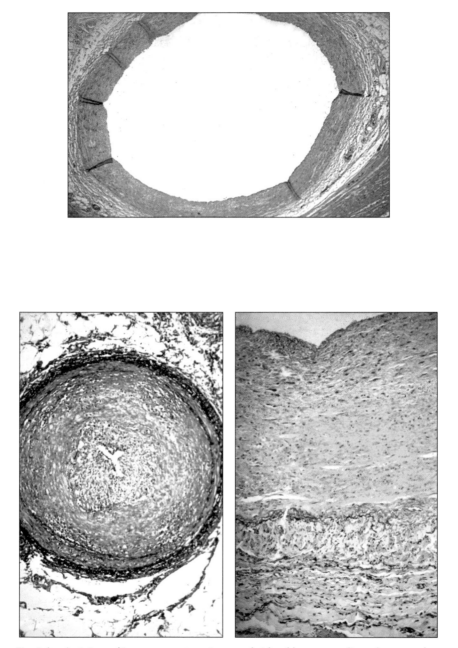

Fig. 3 (top). A "mural" coronary artery, i.e., one bridged by myocardium does not show physiological intimal thickening (LAD, H&E X 40).

Fig. 4 (lower left). Markedly severe obliterative coronary intimal thickening with normal internal elastic membrane and without atherosclerosis. Transplanted heart in situ 202 days (Verhoeff elastic X 50).

Fig. 5 (lower right). Obliterative intimal thickening in a three year old aortocoronary venous bypass graft from a 63 year old woman (Movat X 100).

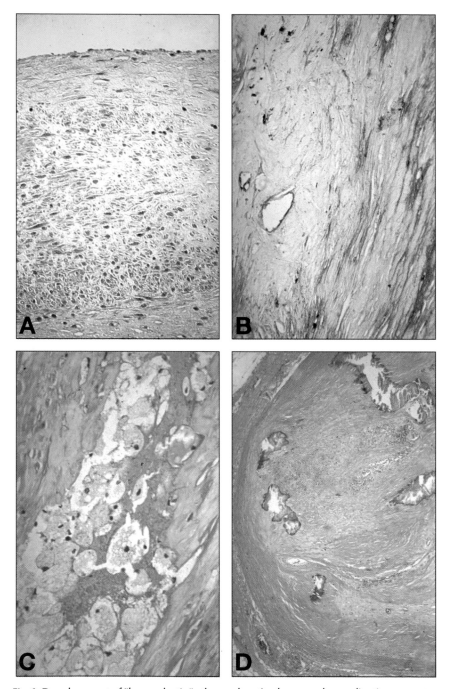

Fig. 6. Development of "hyperplastic" atherosclerotic plaque and complications—see text. (A) Nodular smooth muscle cell hyperplasia in an early plaque without evidence of subendothelial foam cells, cholesterol clefts, platelet aggregates, macrophages or mono-cyte infiltrates. It progresses to the fibrotic, nodular plaque illustrated here (H&E X 100). (B) Proteoglycan accumulation deep in the fibrotic intima (Movat X 250). (C) Foam cells and cholesterol clefts in the proteoglycan pool (H&E X 350). (D) Calcification (H&E X 20);

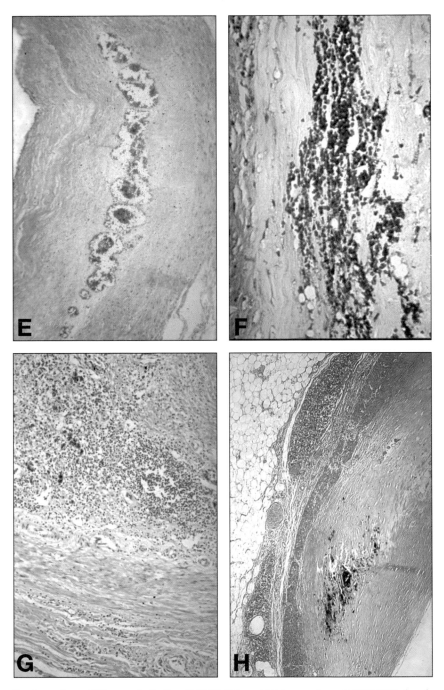

Fig. 6-continued (E) vascularization (H&E X 20) and (F) hemorrhage (H&E X 20) develop in plaques as complications. (G) Adventitial lymphocytic and plasma cell infiltration. This inflammatory reaction begins simultaneously with proteoglycan accumulation in a plaque. In this case (H) it is associated with a semilunar plaque causing minimal lumen stenosis. Note disposition of inflammatory elements around nerves (H&E X 50).

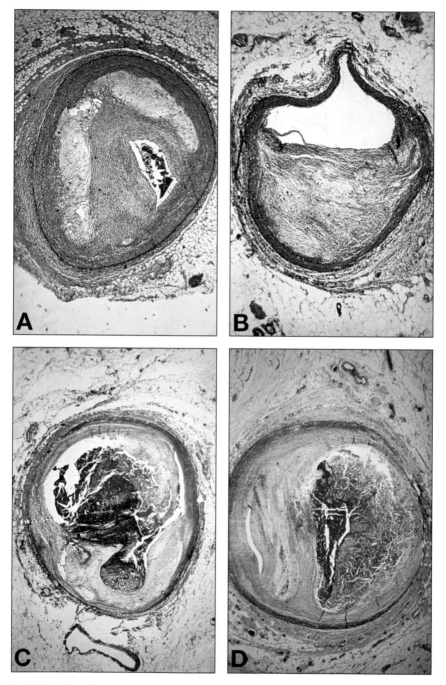

Fig. 7.-Continued on next page.

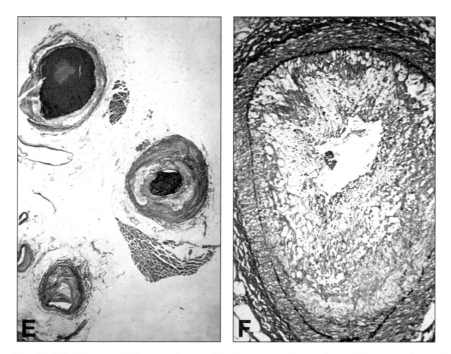

Fig. 7. (A) Advanced fibrous plaque showing smooth muscle cell hyperplasia and proteoglycan accumulation (Movat X19). (B) Semilunar plaque with 50% luminal stenosis. Compliance of the normal arterial wall may produce an almost normal or irregular angiographic image (Movat X20). (C) Intimal rupture or fissuring with small subintimal hemorrhage. Vessel lumen, to left of photograph, filled with thrombus (H&E X100). (D) Histologic section further downstream from C, showing subendothelial hemorrhage and admixture of platelet aggregates and blood clot containing cholesterol crystals in lumen (Movat X13). (E) Three different sections of the same LAD showing an almost normal lumen filled by a coagulum (top); severely reduced lumen occluded by an acute thrombus (middle) and severe semilunar stenosis with empty residual lumen (bottom) (Movat X 15). A pathologist's diagnosis may be altered by the level of section, stressing the importance of step sections through an area of luminal occlusion. Equally, to evaluate flow dynamics in a plaque, all variations in lumen reduction along its course, type of occlusion and collaterals should be considered. (F) "Hypercholesterol" plaque. It is mainly formed by foam cells. This plaque is found in animals following experimental cholesterol diet and in human familial hyperlipidemia. Its progression is different and likely linked to early endothelial damage, subendothelial lipoprotein/cholesterol deposition and monocytic macrophage-reaction (inflammation?); 35 year old man with Type A hyperlipidemia (Weigert elastic X 20). Figs. C & E reprinted with permission from Baroldi G. In: Silver MD, ed. Cardiovascular Pathology, 2nd Ed. New York: Churchill Livingstone Inc.,1991a:487.

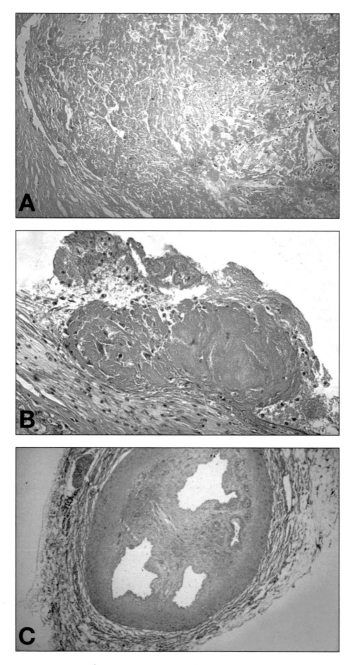

Fig. 8.-Continued on next page.

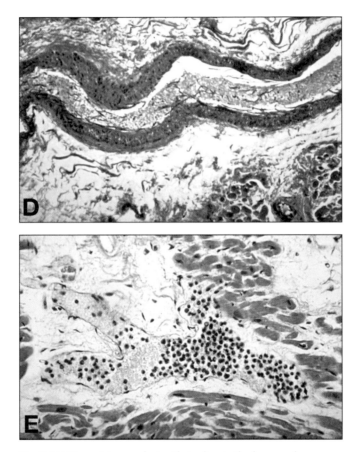

Fig. 8. (A) Organizing occlusive thrombus in the lumen of a coronary artery with newly formed vessels filled by radiopaque material injected postmortem. These small vessels may give an angiographic "blush" clinically (H&E X 100). (B) Organizing mural, platelet-fibrin thrombus (H&E X100). (C) Organized thrombus with recanalization beyond area of maximal lumen stenosis caused by atherosclerosis(H&E X 20). (D) Intramural coagulum formed mainly by red cells (H&E X100). When cessation of blood flow is slow, layering of blood elements occurs. (E) Layering of leukocytes in a vein (H&E X 120).

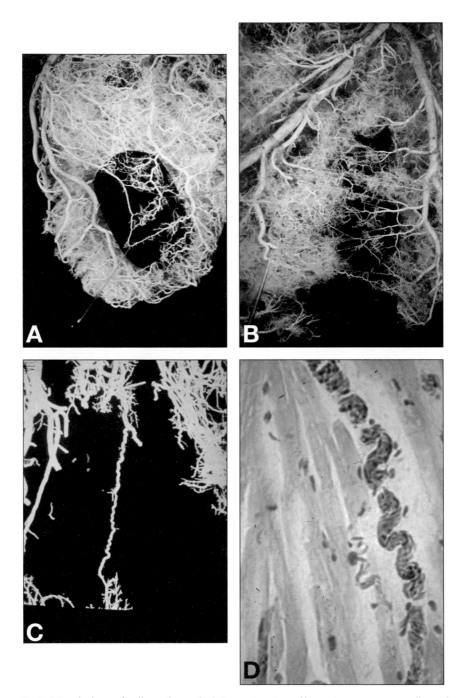

Fig. 9. Morphology of collateral vessels, (A) anterior view of heart. Intercoronary collaterals join LAD with branches of RCA; (B) Homocoronary collaterals between branches of LAD on anterior surface of heart. (C) Typical "corkscrew" appearance of many collaterals. (D) Histologic equivalent of C (H&E x180). The "corkscrew" morphology is likely related to collateral vessel disposition parallel to the line of myocardial contraction. Normal collaterals are part of the terminal bed. Reprinted with permission from Baroldi G. In: Silver MD, ed. Cardiovascular Pathology, 2nd Ed. New York: Churchill Livingstone Inc.,1991a:487.

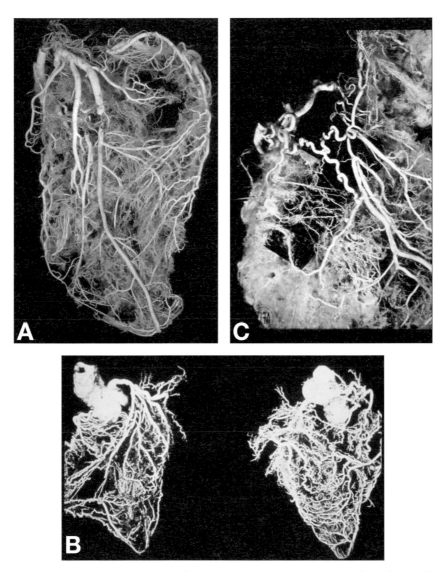

Fig. 10. Any time there is severe lumen reduction of any nature, collaterals (satellite collaterals) increase in size. (A) Occlusion of LAD at origin of first diagonal branch with acute myocardial infarction. Note satellite collaterals angling from RCA to LAD distal to occlusion. (B) Anterior and posterior view of cast of coronary arteries showing double occlusion of LAD and occlusion of RCA. Note satellite collaterals have allowed filling of the whole coronary system. (62 year old man: brain hemorrhage without clinical or postmortem evidence of ischemic heart disease). (C) Large collaterals from LCX to distal tract of an occluded LAD in a 70 year old woman with old and recent myocardial infarcts. Note the numerous normal and not enlarged collaterals in the same area. This indicates that ischemia, per se, is not the cause of collateral enlargement otherwise a diffuse enlargement in the whole ischemic zone might be expected.

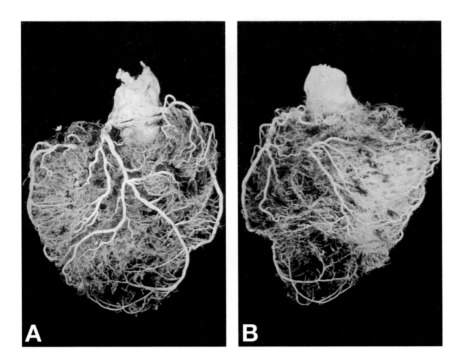

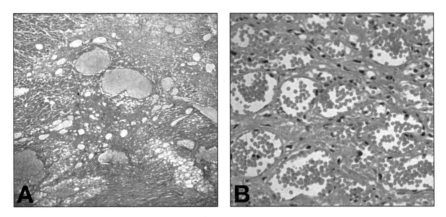

Fig. 11 (top). Anterior (A) and posterior (B) views of coronary artery casts showing a large avascular area of the left apico-posterior ventricle. This corresponds to an infarct. The disappearance of all intramural vessels including collaterals will result in further enlargement of preserved anastomoses (persistence of pressure gradient due to pre existing severe coronary stenosis). Note that the infarcted zone corresponds to a LAD with a practically normal lumen. The occlusion is present in the RCA and "compensated" by collaterals. No infarct in the territory of RCA. How many times in gross dissection do pathologists miss a correct topographical relationship between an occluded coronary artery and a myocardial infarct?

Fig. 12 (bottom). Angiomatous plexus formed by giant capillaries (collaterals) in region of (A) acute infarct (H&E X 50); and (B) scar at old infarct site (H&E X 150).

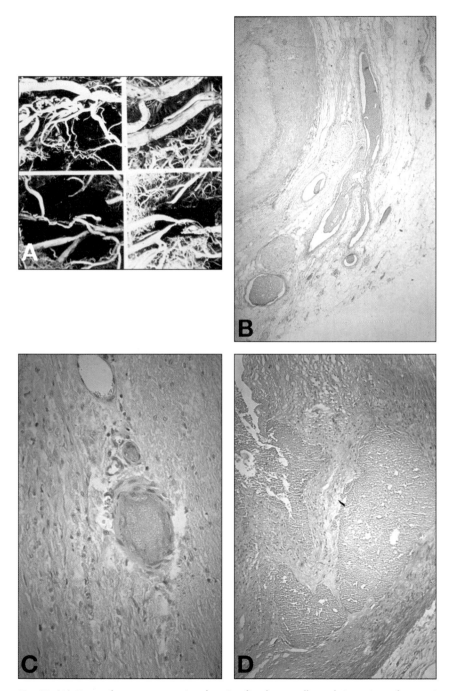

Fig. 13. (A) Casts of coronary arteries showing fine bore collaterals in region of stenosing atherosclerotic plaques They are in the vessel wall. A serial section study done in another series following postmortem injection (unpublished) show vascular connections be-tween adventitial arteries; (B) intimal arterioles in plaque and (C) the residual vascular lumen. Angiomatous-like plexuses (D) that are joined to the residual lumen are also found in the intima. The presence of these intraplaque collaterals make angiographic interpre-tation difficult (H&E X 100). (Fig. A reprinted from Baroldi G 1991a with permission.)

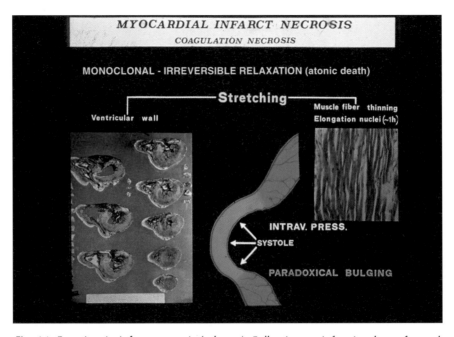

Fig. 14. Function in infarct necrosis (schema). Following an infarction loss of muscle contraction in the infarcted area occurs within a few seconds. Myocells in flaccid paralysis become passive elements stretched by intraventricular pressure. Necrotic myocells show hyperdistended sarcomeres and elongation of nuclei; a pattern visible within 1 hour of experimental coronary occlusion (H&E X 250).

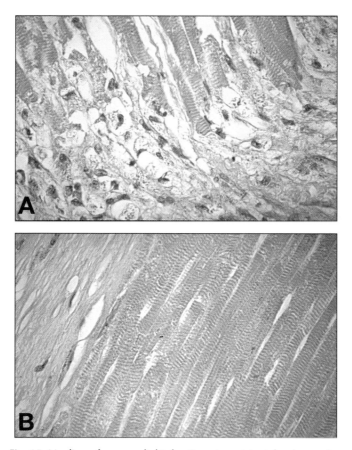

Fig. 15. Healing of myocardial infarction. A centripetal polymorphonuclear infiltration occurs from the periphery of an infarct. This
reaction begins approximately 6 hours from onset, increases in the
next 4 days, with an abscess-like pattern possible in the largest infarcts.
The infiltration is associated with minor fibrin exudation and disap-
pears by lysis of leukocytes within the first week (not illustrated). (A)
Removal of necrotic tissue is accomplished by macrophages (H&E X
400) and followed by fibrosis. (B) The latter shows that in a myocardial
infarction the registered order of distended sarcomeres may be
maintained (to left of photograph) even when scarring is practically
complete (to right of photograph) (H&E X 400).

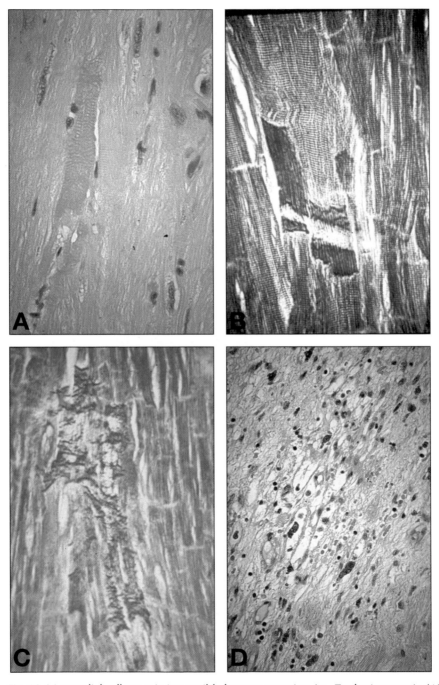

Fig. 16. Myocardial cell arrest in irreversible hypercontraction, i.e., Zenker's necrosis. (A) The first change is hypercontraction of the whole myocell which becomes highly eosinophilic (H&E X 400); (B) Early fragmentation of hypercontracted myocell (PTHA X 400). (C) Total destruction of the contractile apparatus with irregular crossband formation (PTHA X 250). (D) Healing phase with macrophages and collagenization of empty sarcolemmal tubes producing an alveolar pattern (H&E X 250).

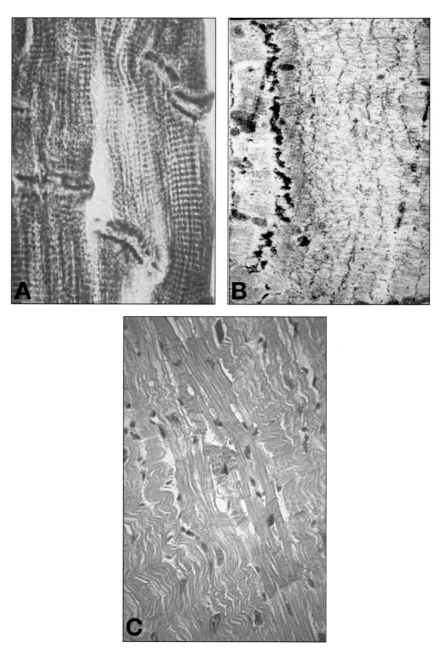

Fig. 17. (A) Hypercontraction of relatively few sarcomeres adjacent to an intercalated disc produces a "paradiscal lesion" seen on one or both sides of a disc, the rest of the myocell being normal (PTHA X 640). (B) "Clear" paradiscal band (EM X 3,500). These different morphologies without myofibrillar rhexis (most of the myocell functions normally) suggest a possible reversible change. Paradiscal lesions are detectable after 5minutes and total or pancellular destruction, after 10-15 minutes following intravenous infusion of noradrenaline. (C) The hypercontraction produces a scalloped sarcolemma and waviness of adjacent normal myocells (H&E X 400). (Figs. A & B reprinted from Baroldi G 1991b with permission.)

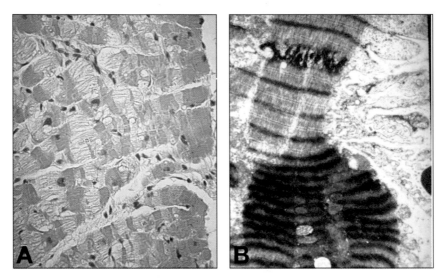

Fig. 18. (A) "Cut edge" lesion in a human heart excised at heart transplantation (H&E X 250). (B) Electron microscopy reveals extremely thickened Z lines and shorting of sarcomeres without myofibrillar rhexis (EM X 5,200). This type of lesion is also found at the edge of endomyocardial biopsies and in either setting is not caused by ischemia.

Fig. 19. Progressive reduction of myocardial function. "Failing death" or colliquative myocytolysis. (A) Mild loss of myofibrils in transverse section producing an alveolar pattern (H&E X 600). (B) Total disappearance of myofibrils in transverse section (H&E X 100). Note there is no inflammatory reaction associated with this change. It may be reversible.

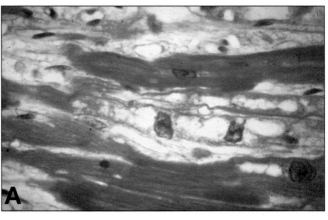

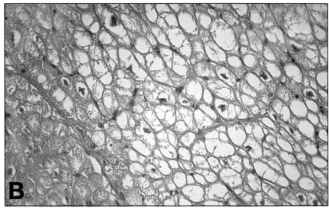

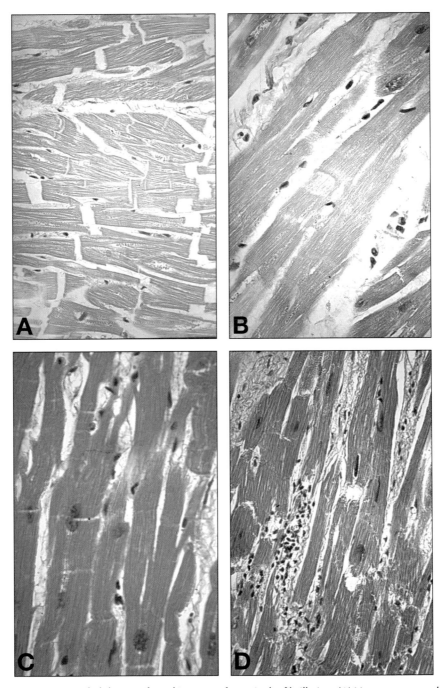

Fig. 20. Myocardial damage found in cases of ventricular fibrillation. (A) Hypercontracted and segmented myocells. Is this really an artifact as many pathologists now believe? (H&E X 400) (B) Widened or stretched discs in hypercontracted myocardium (H&E X 400). (C) Fragmentation dividing a nucleus of the myocell (H&E X 400). (D) Comparable change in sudden and unexpected death in patients with silent Chagas disease (H&E X 400).

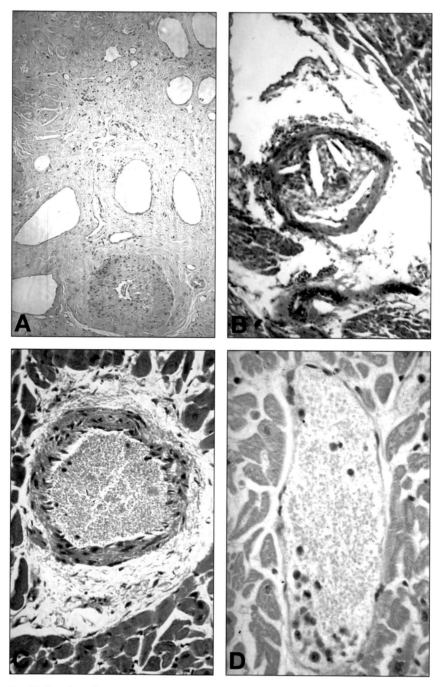

Fig. 21-Continued on next page.

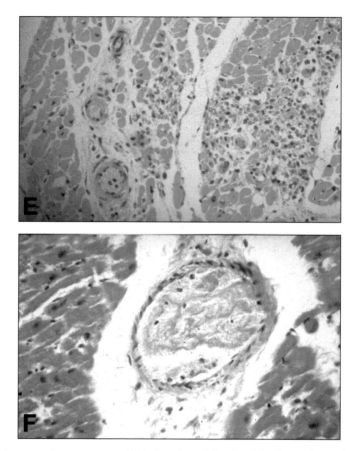

Fig. 21. Intramural coronary arterial lesions in sudden death/ ischemic heart disease. (A) Small arteries with medial hyperplasia and/or intimal thickening or with fibrotic walls related to scar following myocardial infarction (H&E X 100). (B) Atheromatous embolus in a small intramural arteriole with normal surrounding myocardium. This was the only such embolus found in all cases we studied with an average of 40 transmural sections for each heart. (C) Platelet aggregate filling the lumen of an intramural arteriole in a normal subject (H&E X 100). (D) Intramural arteriole filled with platelet aggregate in a woman with angina pectoris who died suddenly. (E) Note healing Zenker necrosis in myocardium of that patient (H&E X 50). (F) Fibrin-platelet aggregates in a patient who died suddenly during angioplasty (H&E X 100).

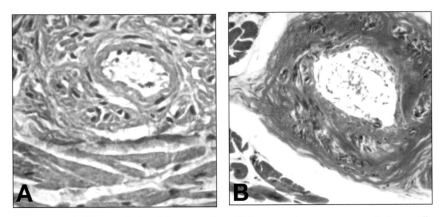

Fig. 22. Medial hyperplasia obliterans of small intramural coronary vessels in papillary muscles, trabeculae carneae or interventricular septum of a normal subject. (A) Thickening of the media mainly by longitudinal smooth muscle cell bundles without intimal thickening (H&E X 150). (B) With time the hyperplastic vessels become fibrotic and may show intimal thickening (Mallory trichrome X 150).

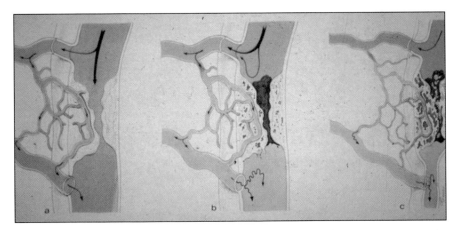

Fig. 23. Schema showing (a) coronary artery stenosis bypassed and compensated for by collaterals. Following a myocardial infarction (b) there is increased peripheral resistance in this area with a progressive blockage of flow causing hemorrhage in the plaque and thrombus formation; (c) coronary artery spasm with plaque rupture, hemorrhage and luminal thrombosis. Reprinted with permission from Baroldi G. In: Silver MD, ed. Cardiovascular Pathology, 2nd Ed. New York: Churchill Livingstone Inc.,1991a:487.

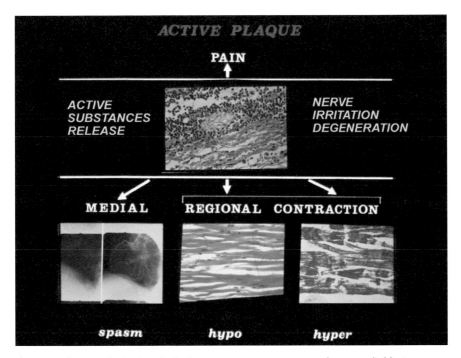

Fig. 24. Schema relating "active" plaque to coronary artery and myocardial lesions—see text. Reprinted with permission from Baroldi G. In: Silver MD, ed. Cardiovascular Pathology, 2nd Ed. New York: Churchill Livingstone Inc., 1991b:643.

REFERENCES

Ablad B. Beta adrenergic mechanisms and atherogenesis. In Hypertension -The tip of an iceberg. Manchester: Adis Press, 1988:23.

Adam RD. Diseases of muscle. In A study in pathology. London: Harper & Row, 1975:452

Adelson L, Hoffman W. Sudden death from coronary disease related to a lethal mechanism arising independently of vascular occlusion or myocardial damage. JAMA 1961; 176:129.

Ahrens PJ, Sheehan FH, Dahl J et al. Extension of hypokinesia into angiographically perfused myocardium in patients with acute infarction. J Am Coll Cardiol 1993; 22:1010.

Aldridge HE, Trimble AS. Progression of proximal coronary artery lesions to total occlusion after aorta-coronary saphenous vein by pass grafting. J Thorac Cardiov Surg 1971; 62:7.

Algra A, Tijssen JGP, Roelandt JRTC et al. Heart rate variability from 24-hour electrocardiography and the 2-year risk for sudden death. Circulation 1993; 88:180.

Alonzo DR, Starek PK, Minick CR. Induction of atherosclerosis in transplanted rabbit hearts by the synergy of graft rejection and cholesterol-rich diet. Circulation 1993; 42 (Suppl 3):5.

Ambrose JA. Plaque disruption and the acute coronary syndromes of unstable angina and myocardial infarction: if the substrate is similar why is the clinical presentation different? J Am Coll Cardiol 1992; 19:1653.

Ambrose JA, Tannenbaum MA, Alexopoulos D et al. Angiographic progression of coronary artery disease and the development of myocardial infarction. J Am Coll Cardiol 1988; 12:56.

Ambrose JA, Winters SL, Arora RR et al.Coronary angiographic morphology in myocardial infarction: a link between the pathogenesis of unstable angina and myocardial infarction. J Am Coll Cardiol 1985a;6:1233.

Ambrose JA, Winters SL, Stern A et al. Angiographic morphology and pathogenesis of unstable angina pectoris. J Am Coll Cardiol 1985b;5:609.

Amsterdam EA, Pan H, Rendig SV et al. Limitation of myocardial infarct size in pigs with a dual lipoxygenase-cyclooxygenase blocking agent by inhibition of neutrophil activity without reduction of neutrophil migration. J Am Coll Cardiol 1993; 22:1738.

Anderson JL, Rodier HE, Green LS. Comparative effects of beta-adrenergic blocking drugs on experimental ventricular fibrillation threshold. Am J Cardiol 1983; 51:1196.

Anderson KP, Stinson EB, Derby GC et al. Vulnerability of patients with obstructive hypertrophic cardiomyopathy to ventricular arrhythmia induction in the operating room. Am J Cardiol 1983; 51:812.

Angelini A, Benciolini P, Thiene G. Radiation-induced coronary obstructive atherosclerosis and sudden death in a teenager. Inter J Cardiol 1985; 9:371.

Angelini A, Thiene G, Frescura G et al. Coronary arterial wall and atherosclerosis in youth (1-20 years): a histologic study in northern Italian population. Intern J Cardiol 1990; 28:361.

Araie E, Fujita M, Ejiri M et al. Relation between the preexistent coronary collateral circulation and recanalization rate of intracoronary thrombolysis for acute myocardial infarction. J Am Coll Cardiol 1990; 15:218A.

Arani DT, Greene DG, Bunnel IL et al. Reductions in coronary flow under resting conditions in collateral dependent myocardium of patients with complete occlusion of the left anterior descending coronary artery. J Am Coll Cardiol 1984; 3:668.

Arbustini E, Grasso M, Diegoli M et al. Coronary atherosclerotic plaques with and without thrombus in ischemic heart syndromes: a morphologic, immunohistochemical and biochemical study. Am J Cardiol 1991; 68:36B.

Ashraf M, White F, Bloor CM. Ultrastructural influence of reperfusing dog myocardium with calcium-free blood after coronary artery occlusion. Am J Pathol 1978; 90:423.

Baba N, Bashe WJ, Keller MD et al. Pathology of atherosclerotic heart disease in sudden death. Organizing thrombosis and acute coronary vessel lesions. Circulation 1975; 53(Suppl 3);51.

Barber MJ, Mueller TM, Henry DP et al. Transmural myocardial infarction in the dog produces sympathectomy in noninfarcted myocardium. Circulation 1983; 67:787.

Barger AC, Beeuwkes R, Lainey LL et al. Hypothesis: Vasa vasorum and neovascularization of human coronary arteries. A possible role in the pathophysiology of atherosclerosis. N Engl J Med 1984; 310:175.

Barnes AR, Ball RG. The incidence and situation of myocardial infarction in one thousand consecutive postmortem examination. Am J Med Sc 1932; 183:215.

Baroldi G. Acute coronary occlusion as a cause of myocardial infarct and sudden coronary heart death. Am J Cardiol 1965; 16:859.

Baroldi G. High resistance of the human myocardium to shock and red blood cell aggregation (sludge). Cardiologia 1969; 54:271.

Baroldi G. The coronary arteries in cor pulmonale. Acta Cardiol 1971a;26:602.

Baroldi G. Functional morphology of the anastomotic circulation in human cardiac pathology. Meth Achievm exp Path 1971b;5:438.

Baroldi G. Different types of myocardial necrosis in coronary heart disease: a pathophysiological review of their functional significance. Am Heart J 1975; 89:742.

Baroldi G. Coronary thrombosis: facts and beliefs. Am Heart J 1976; 91:683.

Baroldi G. Coronary stenosis: ischemic or non ischemic factor? Am Heart J 1978; 96:139.

Baroldi G. The coronary circulation in man. In: Schwartz CJ, Wherthesse NT, Wolf S, eds. Structure and Function of the Circulation. Vol. 2. New York: Plenum Press, 1981:77.

Baroldi G. Limitation of infarct size: Theoretical aspects. In: Chazov EI, Smirnov VN, Organov RG, eds.Cardiology. An International Perspective. Vol. I. New York: Plenum Press, 1984:517.

Baroldi G. Morpho-pathological contribution to the modern interpretation of ischemic heart disease. In: Lenzi S, Deschovich G, eds. (V Intern Symposium of Atherosclerosis, Bologna, Italy 1983). Lancaster: MTP Press, 1985a:279.

Baroldi G. Pathology and mechanisms of sudden death. In: Hurst JW, ed. The Heart. 6th ed. New York: McGraw-Hill Book Co, 1985b:529.

Baroldi G. Medial hyperplasia obliterans of the intramural coronary arterial vessels. G Ital Cardiol 1986; 16:537.

Baroldi G. Diseases of the extramural coronary arteries. In: Silver MD, ed. Cardiovascular Pathology, 2nd Edition. New York: Churchill Livingstone Inc., 1991a:487.

Baroldi G. Morphologic forms of myocardial necrosis related to myocardial cell function. In: Silver MD, ed. Cardiovascular Pathology. 2nd Edition. New York: Churchill Livingstone Inc., 1991b:643.

Baroldi G, Falzi G, Mariani F. Sudden coronary death. A postmortem study in 208 selected cases compared to 97 "control" subjects. Am Heart J 1979; 98:20.

Baroldi G, Falzi G, Mariani F et al. Morphology, frequency and significance of intramural arterial lesions in sudden coronary death. G Ital Cardiol 1980; 10:644.

Baroldi G, Manion WC. Microcirculatory disturbances and human myocardial infarction. Am Heart J 1967; 74:171.

Baroldi G, Marzilli M, L'Abbate A et al. Coronary occlusion: cause or consequence of acute myocardial infarction? A case report. Clin Cardiol 1990; 13,49.

Baroldi G, Milam JD, Wakasch DC et al. Myocardial cell damage in "stone heart". J Mol Cell Cardiol 1974; 6:395.

Baroldi G, Parravicini C, Gaiera G. Sudden cardiac death in a "silent" case of acquired immunodeficiency syndrome (AIDS). G Ital Cardiol 1993; 23:353.

Baroldi G, Radice F, Schmidt C et al. Morphology of acute myocardial infarction in relation to coronary thrombosis. Am Heart J 1974; 87:65.

Baroldi G, Scomazzoni G. Coronary Circulation. in the Normal and Pathologic Heart. American Registry of Pathology, A.F.I.P., ed. Washington DC: U.S. Government Printing Office, 1967.

Baroldi G, Silver MD. The healing of myocardial infarcts in man. Giorn It Cardiol 1975; 5:465.

Baroldi G, Silver MD, Lixfield W et al. Irreversible myocardial damage resembling catecholamine necrosis secondary to acute coronary occlusion in dogs: its prevention by propranolol. J Molec Cell Cardiol 1977; 9:687.

Baroldi G, Silver MD, Mariani F et al. Correlation of morphological variables in the coronary atherosclerotic plaque with clinical patterns of ischemic heart disease. Am J Cardiov Path 1988; 2:159.

Barry JM, Roberts WC, McAllister HA et al. Sudden death in young athletes. Circulation 1980; 62:2.

Basuk WL, Reimer KA, Jennings RB. Effect of repetitive brief episodes of ischemia on cell volume, electrolytes and ultrastructure. J Am Coll Cardiol 1986; 8:33A.

Batsakis JG. Degenerative lesions of the heart. In: Gould SE ed. The Pathology of the Heart and Blood Vessels. 3rd ed. Springfield, Ill.: Charles C Thomas, 1968:479.

Bayés de Luna A, Coumel P, Leclercq JF. Ambulatory sudden cardiac death: mechanisms of production of fatal arrhythmia on the basis of data from 157 cases. Am Heart J 1989; 117:15.

Bayés de Luna A, J Guindo. Sudden death in ischemic heart disease. Rev Port Cardiol 1990b;9(5):473.

Bayés de Luna A, J Guindo, Borja M et al. Recasting the approach to the treatment of potentially malignant ventricular arrhythmias after the CAST study. Cardiov Drugs Ther 1990a;4:651.

Bean WB. Bullet wound of the heart with coronary artery ligation. Am Heart J 1944; 21:375.

Beck CS, Leighninger DS. Hearts too good to die: our problem. Ohio Med J 1960; 56:1221.

Bedford THB. The pathology of sudden death: a review of 198 cases "brought in dead". J Path Bact 1933; 36:333.

Bemis CE, Gorlin R, Kemp HG et al. Progression of coronary artery disease. A clinical arteriographic study. Circulation 1973; 47:455.

Benditt EP. Evidence for a monoclonal origin of human atherosclerotic plaques and some implications. Circulation 1974; 50:650.

Benshop RJ, Nieuwhenhuis EES, Tromp BA et al. Effects of β-adrenergic blockade on immunologic and cardiovascular changes induced by mental stress. Circulation 1994; 89:762.

Berry W. The unsettling of American culture and agriculture. San Francisco, Calif: Sierra Club Books, 1977.

Bertrand ME, LaBlanche JM, Tilmant P et al. Frequency of provoked coronary arterial spasm in 1089 consecutive patients undergoing coronary arteriography. Circulation 1982; 65:1299.

Bieber CP, Stinson EB, Shumway NE et al. Cardiac transplantation in man. VII Pathology. Am J Cardiol 1970; 25:84.

Billingham ME. The postsurgical heart. The pathology of cardiac transplantation. Am J Cardiov Path 1988; 1:319.

Bing RJ, Tillmanns H, Fauvel JM et al. Effect of prolonged alcohol administration on calcium transport in heart muscle of the dog. Circ Res 1974; 35:33.

Bishop YMM, Fienberg SE, Holland PW. Discrete multivariate analysis, 6th ed. Cambridge, Mass: MIT Press, 1980.

Black A, Black MM, Gensini G et al. Exertion and acute coronary artery injury. Circulation 1965; 32 (Suppl 2):3.

Blake HA, Manion WC, Mattingly TW et al. Coronary artery anomalies. Circulation 1964:30:927.

Bloom S, Cancilla DA. Myocytolysis and mitochondrial calcification in rat myocardium after low doses of isoproterenol. Am J Pathol 1969; 54:373.

Blumgart HL, Schlesinger MJ, Davis D. Studies on the relation of the clinical manifestations of angina pectoris, coronary thrombosis and myocardial infarction to the pathologic findings with particular reference to the significance of the collateral circulation. Am Heart J 1940; 19:1.

Bodenheimer MM, Banka VS, Hermann GA et al. Reversible asynergy: histopathologic and electrographic correlations in patients with coronary artery disease. Circulation 1976; 3:792.

Bodenheimer MM, Banka VS, Hermann GA et al. The effect of severity of coronary artery obstructive disease and the coronary collateral circulation on local histopathologic and electrographic observations in man. Am J Med 1977; 63:193.

Bolli R, Zhu W, Thornby JI et al. Time course and determinants of recovery of function after reversible ischemia in conscious dogs. Am J Physiol 1988; 254:H102.

Bonow RO, Quyyumi AA, Panza JA et al. Do repeated episodes of reversible myocardial ischemia lead to progressive left ventricular dysfunction in mildly symptomatic patients with coronary artery disease? J Am Coll Cardiol 1990; 15:203A.

Borgers M, Thoné F, Wouters L et al. Structural correlates of regional myocardial dysfunction in patients with critical coronary stenosis: chronic hibernation? Cardiovasc Pathol 1993; 2:237.

Bork K. Ueber die Kranzadersklerose. Virchow Arch Path Anat 1926; 262:646.

Born GVR, Honour AJ, Mitchell JRA. Inhibition by adenosine and by 2-chloroadenosine of the formation and embolization of platelet thrombi. Nature 1964; 4934:761.

Bouchardy B, Majno G. A new approach to the histologic diagnosis of early myocardial infarcts. Cardiology 1971-72;56:327.

Boyd W. In: A Textbook of Pathology: Structure and Function In Disease. 7th ed. Philadelphia: Lea & Febiger, 1961:196.

Bradbury S. Thirty years after ligation of the anterior descending branch of the left coronary artery. Am Heart J 1942; 24:562.

Brain MC, Dacie JV, Hourihane DOB. Microangiopathic haemolytic anaemia: the possible role of vascular lesions in pathogenesis. Brit J Haemat 1962; 8:358.

Brandenburg RO. Cardiomyopathies and their role in sudden death. J Am Coll Cardiol 1985; 5:185B.

Branwood AW, Montgomery GL. Observations on the morbid anatomy of coronary artery disease. Scottish M.J 1956; 1:376.

Braunwald E, Kloner RA. The stunned myocardium: prolonged, postischemic ventricular dysfunction. Circulation 1982; 66:1146.

Braunwald E, Rutherford JD. Reversible ischemic left ventricular dysfunction: evidence for the "hibernating myocardium". J Am Coll Cardiol 1986; 8:1467.

Brechenmacher C, Coumel P, Fauchier JP et al. De Subitaneis Mortibus. XXII. Intractable paroxysmal tachycardias which proved fatal in type A Wolff-Parkinson-White Syndrome. Circulation 1977; 55:408.

Brechenmacher C, Coumel P, James TN. De Subitaneis Mortibus. XVI. Intractable tachycardia in infancy. Circulation 1976; 53:377.

Bridges JM, Weaver JA. Platelet stickness. Am Heart J 1966; 71:291.

Brody WR, Angeli WW, Kosek JC. Histologic fate of the venous coronary artery bypass in dogs. Am J Path 1972; 66:111.

Brouardel F, Benham FL. Death and Sudden Death. NY:William Wood Co, 1902.

Brown G, Albers JJ, Fisher LD et al. Regression of coronary artery disease as a result of intensive lipid-lowering therapy in men with high levels of apolipoprotein. B. N Engl J Med 1990; 323:1289.

Brown GB, Gallery CA, Badger RS et al. Incomplete lysis of thrombus in the moderate underlying atherosclerotic lesion during intracoronary infusion of streptokinase for acute myocardial infarction: quantitative angiographic observations. Circulation 1986; 73:653.

Buja ML, Poliner LR, Parkey RW et al. Clinicopathologic study of persistently positive technetium-99 stannous pyrophosphate myocardial scintigrams and myocytolytic degeneration after myocardial infarction. Circulation 1977; 56:1016.

Buja ML, Willerson JT. Clinicopathologic correlates of acute ischemic heart disease syndromes. Am J Cardiol 1981; 47:343.

Buja ML, Willerson JT. Role of inflammation in coronary plaque disruption. Circulation 1994; 89:503.

Bulkley BH, Hutchins GM. Accelerated "atherosclerosis". A morphologic study of 97 saphenous vein coronary artery bypass grafts. Circulation 1977; 55:163.

Bulkley BH, Klacsmann PG, Hutchins GM. Angina pectoris, myocardial infarction and sudden cardiac death with normal coronary arteries: a clinicopathologic study of 9 patients with progressive systemic sclerosis. Am Heart J 1978; 95:563.

Burch GE, De Pasquale NP. Arteriosclerosis in high pressure and low pressure coronary arteries. Am Heart J 1962; 63:720.

Burke AP, Subramanian R, Smialek J et al. Nonatherosclerotic narrowing of the atrioventricular node artery and sudden death. J Am Coll Cardiol 1993; 21:117.

Burns CJ, Manion WC. Sudden unexpected death of a two-year-old child from thrombosis of both coronary arteries with aneurysmal dilatation of the vessels. Med Ann District of Columbia 1969; 38:381.

Burton AC. Relation of structure to function of the tissues of the wall of blood vessels. Physiol Rev 1954; 34:619.

Cabin HS, Clubb KS, Vita N et al. Regional dysfunction by equilibrium radionuclide angiocardiography: a clinicopathologic study evaluating the relation of degree of dysfunction to the presence and extent of myocardial infarction. J Am Coll Cardiol 1987; 4:743.

Calkins H, Allman K, Bolling S et al. Correlation between scintigraphic evidence of regional sympathetic neuronal dysfunction and ventricular refractoriness in the human heart. Circulation 1993; 89:172.

Cannon WB. "Voodoo" death. Am Anthropol 1942; 44:169.

Carleton RA, Boyd T. Traumatic laceration of the anterior coronary artery treated by ligation without myocardial infarction: report of a case with a review of the literature. Am Heart J 1958; 56:136.

Carlson RE, Schott RJ, Buda AJ. Neutrophil depletion fails to modify myocardial no reflow and functional recovery after coronary reperfusion. J Am Coll Cardiol 1989; 7:1803.

Carroll SM, White FC, Roth DM et al. Heparin accelerates coronary collateral development in a porcine model of coronary artery occlusion. Circulation 1993; 88:198.

Cebelin MS, Hirsch CS. Human stress cardiomyopathy. Myocardial lesions in victims of homicidal assaults without internal injuries. Hum Path 1980; 11:123.

Chandler AB, Chapman I, Erhardt LR et al. Coronary thrombosis in myocardial infarction. Report of a workshop on the role of coronary thrombosis in the pathogenesis of acute myocardial infarction. Am J Cardiol 1974; 34:823.

Cheitlin MD, De Castro CM, McAllister HA. Sudden death as a complication of anomalous left coronary origin from the anterior sinus of Valsalva. A not-so-minor congenital anomaly. Circulation 1974; 50:780.

Cheng TO, Bashour T, Shing BK et al. Myocardial infarction in the absence of coronary arteriosclerosis. Am J Cardiol 1972; 30:680.

Chesler E, King RA, Edwards JE. The myxomatous mitral valve and sudden death. Circulation 1983; 67:632.

Chilian WM, Mass HJ, Williams SM et al. Microvascular occlusions promote coronary collateral growth. Am J Physiol 258, 1990;(Heart Circ Physiol 27) H1103.

Ciuffo AA, Ouyang P, Becker LC et al. Reduction of sympathetic inotropic response after ischemia in dogs. Contributor to stunned myocardium. J Clin Invest 1985; 75:1504.

Claudon DG, Claudon DB, Edwards JE. Primary dissecting aneurysm of coronary artery. A cause of acute myocardial ischemia. Circulation 1972; 45:259.

Cliff WJ, Heathcote CR, Moss NS et al. The coronary arteries in cases of cardiac and non cardiac sudden death. Am J Pathol 1988; 192:319.

Clusin WT, Bristow MR, Karagueuzian HS et al. Do calcium-dependent ionic currents mediate ischemic ventricular fibrillation? Am J Cardiol 1982; 49:606.

Cobb LA, Baum RS, Schaffer WA. Resuscitation from out-of-hospital ventricular fibrillation: 4 years follow-up. Circulation 1975; 51-52(Suppl 3):223.

Cobb LA, Werner JA. Predictors and prevention of sudden cardiac death. In: Hurst JW, ed. The Heart.6th Edition. New York: Mc Graw Hill Book Co, 1986. p538.

Cobb LA, Werner JA, Trobaugh GB. Sudden cardiac death. I A decade's experience with out-of-hospital resuscitation. Modern Concepts Cardiov Dis 1980a;6:31.

Cobb LA, Werner JA, Trobaugh GB. Sudden cardiac death. II Outcome of resuscitation, management and future directions. Modern Concepts Cardiov Dis 1980b;7:37.

Cohen MV. The functional value of coronary collaterals in myocardial ischemia and therapeutic approach to enhance collateral flow. Am Heart J 1978; 95:396.

Cohn LH, Kosek J, Angell WW. Pulmonary arteriosclerosis produced by hyperoxemic normotensive perfusion. Circulation 1970; 42(Suppl 3):114.

Cohn PF. Silent myocardial ischemia and infarction. 2nd ed. New York: Marcel Dekker Inc., 1989.

Cohn PF, Maddox DE, Holman BL et al. Effect of coronary collateral vessels on regional myocardial blood flow in patients with coronary artery disease. Relation of collateral circulation to vasodilator reserve and left ventricular function. Am J Cardiol 1980; 46:359.

Cohnheim J, Schulthess-Rechberg von A. Ueber die Folgen der Kranzarterienverschliessung fur das Herz. Virchow Arch Path Anat 1881; 85:503.

Connor RCR. Focal myocytolysis and fuchsinophilic degeneration of the myocardium of patients dying with various brain lesions. Ann NY Acad Sci 1969; 156:261.

Constantinides P. The role of endothelial injury in arterial thrombosis and atherogenesis. In: Halonen PI, Louhita A, eds. Thrombosis and Coronary Heart Disease. Basel: Karger, Advances in Cardiology 1970:4:67.

Cooley DA, Bloodwell RD, Hallman GL et al. Human cardiac transplantation. Circulation 1969;(Suppl I):1.

Corbalan R, Verrier R, Lown B. Psychological stress and ventricular arrhythmias during myocardial infarction in the conscious dog. Am J Cardiol 1974; 34:692.

Corday E, Heng MK, Meerbaum S et al. Derangements of myocardial metabolism preceding onset of ventricular fibrillation after coronary occlusion. Am J Cardiol 1977; 39:880.

Cowley MJ, Disciascio G, Rehr RB et al. Angiographic observations and clinical relevance of coronary thrombus in unstable angina pectoris. Am J Cardiol 1989; 63:108E.

Cowley MJ, Hastillo A, Vetrovec GW et al. Effects of intracoronary streptokinase in acute myocardial infarction. Am Heart J 1981; 102:1149.

Crawford T, Crawford MD. Prevalence and pathological changes of ischemic heart disease in a hard-water and in a soft-water area. Lancet 1967; 1:229.

Crawford T, Dexter D, Teare RD. Coronary artery pathology in sudden death from myocardial ischemia. Lancet: 1961;Jan 28,181.

Cribier A, Korsatz L, Koning R et al. Improved myocardial ischemic response and enhanced collateral circulation with long repetitive coronary occlusion during angioplasty: a prospective study. J Am Coll Cardiol 1992; 20:578.

Croce L, Noseda V, Bertelli A et al. Sudden and unexpected death from heart disease. Epidemiologic, anatomo- and physiopathologic aspects. A study of 1047 cases. Cardiologia 1960; 37:331.

Cruickshank JM, Pennert K, Sornan AE et al. Low mortality from all causes including myocardial infarction, in well-controlled hypertensives treated with a beta-blocker plus other antihypertensives. J Hypertension 1987; 5:489.

D'Amore PA, Thompson RW. Mechanisms of angiogenesis. Ann Rev Physiol 1987; 49:453.

Davies MJ, Thomas A. Thrombosis and acute coronary artery lesions in sudden cardiac ischemic death. N Engl J Med 1984; 310:1137.

Davies MJ, Thomas AC, Knapman PA et al. Intramyocardial platelet aggregation in patients with unstable angina suffering sudden ischemic cardiac death. Circulation 1986; 73:418.

Davies MJ, Woolf N, Robertson WB. Pathology of acute myocardial infarction with particular reference to occlusive coronary thrombi. Br Heart J 1976; 38:659.

Deutsch E, Berger M, Kussmaul WG et al. Adaptation to ischemia during percutaneous transluminal coronary angioplasty. Clinical, hemodynamic and metabolic features. Circulation 1990; 82:2044.

DeWood MA, Spores J, Notske R et al. Prevalence of total coronary occlusion during the early hours of transmural myocardial infarction. N Engl J Med 1980; 303:897.

DeWood MA, Stifter WF, Simpson CS et al. Coronary arteriographic findings soon after non-Q-wave myocardial infarction. N Engl J Med 1986; 315:417.

Dhurandhar RW, Watt DL, Silver MD et al. Printzmetal's variant form of angina with arteriographic evidence of coronary arterial spasm. Am J Cardiol 1972; 30:902.

Dietz WA, Tobis JM, Isner JM. Failure of angiography to accurately depict the extent of coronary artery narrowing in three fatal cases of percutaneous transluminal coronary angioplasty. J Am Coll Cardiol 1992; 19:1261.

Dock W. The predilection of atherosclerosis for the coronary arteries. JAMA 1946; 131:875.

Donald DE. Myocardial performance after excision of the extrinsic nerves in the dog. Circ Res 1974; 34:417.

Dreyer WJ, Michael LH, West MS et al. Neutrophil accumulation in ischemic canine myocardium: insights into the time course, distribution and mechanism of localization during early reperfusion. Circulation 1991; 84:400.

Duren DR, Becker AE. Focal myocytolysis mimicking the electrocardiographic pattern of transmural anteroseptal myocardial infarction. Chest 1976; 4:506.

Ehrich W, de la Chapelle CE, Cohn AE. Anatomical ontogeny; man; study of coronary arteries. Am J Anat 1931; 49:241.

Eisenberg S. Blood viscosity and fibrinogen concentration following cerebral infarction. Circulation 1966; 33-34 (Suppl 2):10.

El-Maraghi N, Genton E. The relevance of platelet and fibrin thromboembolism of the coronary microcirculation, with special reference to sudden cardiac death. Circulation 1980; 62:936.

Eliot RS. From stress to strength. New York: Bantam Books, 1994

Eliot RS, Baroldi G, Leone A. Necropsy studies in myocardial infarction with minimal or no coronary luminal reduction due to atherosclerosis. Circulation 1974; 49:1127.

Eliot RS, Buell JC. Role of emotions and stress in the genesis of sudden death. J Am Coll Cardiol 1985; 5:95B.

Ellis SG, Henschke CI, Sandor T et al. Time course of functional and bio-
    chemical recovery of myocardium salvaged by reperfusion. J Am Coll Cardiol
    1983; 1:1047.

Emberson JW, Muir AR. Changes in ultrastructure of rat myocardium induced
    by hypokalaemia. J Exp Physiol 1969; 54:36.

Engel G. Sudden and rapid death during psychological stress. Folklore or folk
    wisdom. Ann Int Med 1971; 74:771.

Engler RL, Dahljren MD, Morris DD et al. Role of leukocytes in response to
    acute myocardial ischemia and reflow in dogs. Am J Physiol 1986; 251:H314.

Entman ML, Ballantyne CM. Inflammation in acute coronary syndromes. Cir-
    culation 1993; 88:800.

Entman ML, Hackel DB, Martin AM et al. Prevention of myocardial lesions
    during hemorrhagic shock in dogs by pronethalol. Arch Pathol 1965; 83:392.

Entman ML, Michael LH, Rossen RD et al. Inflammation in the course of
    early myocardial ischemia. FASEB J 1991; 5:2529.

Erhardt LR, Unge G, Boman G. Formation of coronary arterial thrombi in
    relation to onset of necrosis in acute myocardial infarction in man. A clini-
    cal autoradiographic study. Am Heart J 1976; 91:592.

Escaned J, Suylen van RJ, MacLeod DC et al. Histologic characteristic of tissue
    excised during directional coronary atherectomy in stable and unstable an-
    gina pectoris. Am J Cardiol 1993; 71:1442.

Estanol BV, Loyo MV, Mateos HJ et al. Cardiac arrhythmias in experimental
    subarachnoid hemorrhage. Stroke 1977; 8:440.

Esterly JA, Glagow S, Ferguson DJ. Morphogenesis of intimal obliterative
    hyperplasia of small arteries in experimental pulmonary hypertension. An
    ultrastructural study of the role of smooth-muscle cells. Am J Path 1968;
    52:325.

Factor SM. Smooth muscle contraction bands in the media of coronary arter-
    ies: a postmortem marker of antemortem coronary spasm. J Am Coll Cardiol
    1985; 6:1326.

Factor SM, Minase T, Cho S et al. Microvascular spasm in the cardiomyopathic
    Syrian hamster: a preventable cause of focal myocardial necrosis. Circulation
    1982; 66:342.

Falk E. Unstable angina with fatal outcome: dynamic coronary thrombosis lead-
    ing to infarction and/or sudden death. Autopsy evidence of recurrent mural
    thrombosis with peripheral embolization culminating in total vascular occlu-
    sion. Circulation 1985; 71:699.

Falk E. Why do plaques rupture? Circulation 1992; 86 (Suppl 3):3-30.

Falk RH, Rubinow A, Cohen AS. Cardiac arrhythmias in systemic amyloidosis:
    correlation with echocardiographic abnormalities. J Am Coll Cardiol 1984;
    3:107.

Fangman RJ, Hellwig CA. Histology of coronary arteries in newborn infants.
    Am J Path 1947; 23:901.

Farb A, Kolodgie FD, Jenkins M et al. Myocardial infarct extension during
    reperfusion after coronary artery occlusion: pathologic evidence. J Am Coll
    Cardiol 1993; 21:1245.

Faruqui AMA, Maloy WC, Felner JM et al. Symptomatic myocardial bridging of coronary artery. Am J Cardiol 1978; 41:1305.

Ferrans VJ, Buja M, Maron BJ. Myofibrillar abnormalities following cardiac muscle cell injury. In: Fleckstein A, Rona G, eds. Recent Advances in Studies on Cardiac Structure and Metabolism. Vol 6. Baltimore: University Park Press, 1975:367.

Ferrari R, Alfieri O, Curello S et al. Occurrence of oxidative stress during reperfusion of the human heart. Circulation 1990; 8:201.

Fisch C, Armstrong WP, Bigger TJ et al. Sudden Cardiac Death. Clinical electrophysiology and electrocardiography: Summary. J Am Coll Cardiol 1985; 5 (Suppl 6):27B.

Flaherty JT, Pierce JE, Ferrans VJ et al. Endothelial nuclear pattern in the canine arterial tree with particular reference to hemodynamic events. Circul Res 1972; 30:23.

Flameng W, Schwarz F, Hehrlein FW. Intraoperative evaluation of the functional significance of coronary collateral vessels in patients with coronary artery disease. Am J Cardiol 1978; 42:187.

Flameng W, Van Belle H, Vanhaecke J et al. Relation between coronary artery stenosis and myocardial purine metabolism, histology and regional function in humans. J Am Coll Cardiol 1987; 9:1235.

Fleckenstein A, Janke J, Doring HJ et al. Myocardial fiber necrosis due to intracellular Ca^{++} overload. A new principle in cardiac pathophysiology. In: Dhalla NS, ed. Recent Advances in Studies on Cardiac Structure and Metabolism. Vol 4. Baltimore: University Park Press, 1975:563.

Flynn MS, Kern MJ, Donohue TJ et al. Alterations of coronary collateral blood flow velocity during intraaortic balloon pumping. Am J Cardiol 1993; 71:1451.

Folts JD, Gallagher K, Rowe GG. Blood flow reduction in stenosed canine coronary arteries: vasospasm or platelet aggregation? Circulation 1982; 65:248.

Forman MB, Collins W, Kopelman HA et al. Determinants of left ventricular aneurysm formation after anterior myocardial infarction: a clinical and angiographic study. J Am Coll Cardiol 1986; 8:1256.

Forman MD, Oates JA, Robertson D et al. Increased adventitial mast cells in a patient with coronary spasm. N Engl J Med 1985; 313:1138.

Forrester JS, Litvack F, Grundfest W et al. A perspective of coronary disease seen through the arteries of living man. Circulation 1987; 75:505.

Fozzard HA. Electromechanical dissociation and its possible role in sudden cardiac death. J Am Coll Cardiol 1985; 5(Suppl 6):31B.

Franco A. La mort subite due a une maladie du coeur. Arch Mal Coeur 1962; 6:632.

Freifeld AG, Schuster EH, Bulkley BH. Non transmural versus transmural myocardial infarction. A morphological study. Am J Med 1983; 75:423.

French JE, Jennings MA, Poole JCF et al. Intimal changes in the arteries of aging swine. Proc Roy Soc 1962; 158:24.

Friedman M. The coronary canalized thrombus. Provenance, structure function and relationship to death due to coronary artery disease. Brit J Exp Path 1967; 48:556.

Friedman M. The pathogenesis of coronary plaques, thromboses and hemorrhages: an evaluative review. Circulation 1975; 51-52(Suppl 3):34.

Friedman M, Bovenkamp GJ. The pathogenesis of coronary thrombus. Am J
Path 1966; 48:19.

Friedman M, Manwaring JH, Rosenman RH et al. Instantaneous and sudden
deaths. Clinical and pathological differentation in coronary artery disease.
JAMA 1973; 225:1319.

Frink RJ, Trowbridge JO, Roney PA Jr. Nonobstructive coronary thrombosis
in sudden cardiac death. Am J Cardiol 1978; 42:48.

Fry DL. Certain chemorheologic considerations regarding the blood vascular
interface with particular reference to coronary artery disease. Circulation 1969;
40(Suppl 4):38.

Fujita M, Sasayama S, Asanoi H et al. Improvement of treadmil capacity and
collateral circulation as a result of exercise with heparin pretreatment in patients with effort angina. Circulation 1988; 5:1022.

Fujiwara H, Onodera T, Tanaka M et al. A clinicopathologic study of patients
with hemorrhagic myocardial infarction treated with selective thrombolysis
with urokinase. Circulation 1986; 73:749.

Fulton M, Julian DG, Oliver MF. Sudden death and myocardial infarction.
Circulation 1969; 40(Suppl. 4):182.

Fulton WFW. The Coronary Arteries, Microanatomy and Pathogenesis of Obliterative Coronary Artery Disease. Springfield Ill: Charles C. Thomas, 1965.

Fulton WFW, Sumner DJ. Causal role of coronary thrombotic occlusion and
myocardial infarction: evidence of stereoautoradiography serial sections and
1251 fibrinogen autoradiography. Am J Cardiol 1977; 39:322.

Fung AY, Rabkin SW. Beneficial effects of streptokinase on left ventricular function after myocardial reoxygenation and reperfusion following global ischemia
in the isolated rabbit heart. J Cardiovasc Pharmacol 1984; 6:429.

Fuster V, Badimon JJ, Badimon L. Clinical-pathological correlations of coronary disease progression and regression. Circulation 1992; 86 (Suppl 3):31.

Galasssi AR, Crea F, Aranjo LI et al. Comparison of regional myocardial blood
flow in syndrome X and one-vessel coronary artery disease. Am J Cardiol
1993; 72:134.

Ganz W, Buchbinder N, Marcus H et al. Intracoronary thrombolysis in acute
myocardial infarction: experimental background and clinical experience. Am
Heart J 1981; 102:1145.

Gavin JB. The no-reflow phenomenon in ischemic myocardium. Int Rev Exp
Path 1983; 25:361.

Geer JC, McGill HC, Robertson WB et al. Histologic characteristics of coronary artery fatty streaks. Lab Invest 1968; 18:565.

Geft IL, Fishbein MC, Ninomiya K et al. Intermittent brief periods of ischemia
have a cumulative effect and may cause myocardial necrosis. Circulation 1982;
66:1150.

Geiringer E. The mural coronary. Am Heart J 1951a;41:359.

Geiringer E. Intimal vascularization and atherosclerosis. J Path Bact
1951b;63:201.

Gensini GG, Costa BCB. The coronary collateral circulation in living man. Am J Cardiol 1969; 24:393.

Gensini GG, Kelly AE. Incidence and progression of coronary artery disease. An angiographic correlation in 1263 patients. Arch Intern Med 1972; 129:814.

Ghidoni JJ, Liotta D, Thomas H. Massive subendocardial damage accompanying prolonged ventricular fibrillation. Am J Path 1969; 56:15.

Gibbons LW, Cooper KH, Meyer BM et al. The acute cardiac risk of strenuous exercise. JAMA 1980; 244:1799.

Goldstein RE, Borer JS, Epstein SE. Augmentation of contractility following ischemia in the isolated supported heart. Am J Cardiol 1972; 29:265.

Goldstein S. Sudden Death and Coronary Heart Disease. New York: Futura Publ. Co. Inc., 1974.

Goldstein S. The necessity of a uniform definition of sudden coronary death: witnessed death within 1 hour of the onset of acute symptoms. Am Heart J 1982; 103:156.

Goldstein S, Friedman L, Hutchinson R et al. Timing, mechanism and clinical setting of witnessed deaths in postmyocardial infarction patients. J Am Coll Cardiol 1984; 3:1111.

Goldstein S, Landis JR, Leighton R et al. Characteristics of the resuscitated out-of-hospital cardiac arrest victim with coronary heart disease. Circulation 1981; 64:977.

Gomes AJ, Alexopoulos D, Winters SL et al. The role of silent ischemia, the arrhythmic substrate and the short-long sequence in the genesis of sudden cardiac death. J Am Coll Cardiol 1989; 14:1618.

Goodwin JF, Krikler DM. Arrhythmias as a cause of sudden death in hypertrophic cardiomyopathy. Lancet: 1976; 2:927.

Goodwin JF, Krikler DM. Sudden death in cardiomyopathy. In: Manninen V, Halonen PI, eds. Sudden Coronary Death. Basel: Karger, Adv Cardiol 1978; 25:9.

Gorlin R, Fuster V, Ambrose JA. Anatomic-physiologic links between acute coronary syndromes. Circulation 1986; 74:6.

Gotoh K, Minamino T, Katoh O et al. The role of intracoronary thrombus in unstable angina: angiographic assessment and thrombolytic therapy during ongoing anginal attacks. Circulation 1988; 77:526.

Gottlieb A, Masse S, Allard J et al. Concentric hemorrhagic necrosis of the myocardium. A morphological and clinical study. Hum Pathol 1977; 8:27.

Gradman AH, Bell PA, De Busk RF. Sudden death during ambulatory monitoring. Clinical and electrocardiographic correlations. Report of a case. Circulation 1977; 55:210.

Graham AF, Schroeder JS, Rider AK et al. Accelerated atherosclerosis in the human transplanted heart: precipitating factors and possible prevention. Circulation 1972; 46 (Suppl 2):60.

Gravanis MB, Robinson K, Santoian EC et al. The reparative phenomena at the site of balloon angioplasty in human and experimental models. Cardiovasc Pathol 1993; 2:263.

Gregg DE. Coronary Circulation in Health and Disease.Philadelphia: Lea Febiger,1950.

Gregg DE. The natural history of collateral development. Circ Res 1974; 35:335.

Gregg DE, Patterson RE. Functional importance of the coronary collaterals. New Engl J Med 1980; 303:1404.

Griffith LSC, Achuff SC, Conti R at al. Changes in intrinsic coronary circulation and segmental ventricular motion after saphenous-vein coronary bypass graft surgery. New Engl J Med 1973; 288:590.

Gropel RJ, Siegel BA, Perez JE. Recovery of contractile function in viable but dysfunctional myocardium is dependent upon maintenance of oxidative metabolism. J Am Coll Cardiol 1990; 15:203A.

Guthrie RB, Vlodaver Z, Nicoloff DM et al. Pathology of stable and unstable angina pectoris. Circulation 1975; 51:1059.

Habib GB, Heibig J, Forman SA et al. Influence of coronary collateral vessels on myocardial infarct size in humans. Results of phase I thrombolysis in myocardial infarction (TIMI) trial. Circulation 1991; 83:739.

Hackel DB, Reimer KA. Sudden death cardiac and other causes. Durham, NC: Carolina Academic Press, 1993.

Hackett D, Verwilghen J, Davies G et al. Coronary stenoses before and after acute myocardial infarction. Am J Cardiol 1989; 63:1517.

Haerem JW. Platelet aggregates in intramyocardial vessels of patients dying suddenly and unexpectedly of coronary artery disease. Atherosclerosis 1972; 15:199.

Haerem JW. Myocardial lesions in sudden unexpected coronary death. Am Heart J 1975; 90:562.

Haft JI, Al-Zarka AM. Comparison of the natural history of irregular and smooth coronary lesions: insights into the pathogenesis, progression and prognosis of coronary atherosclerosis. Am Heart J 1993; 126:551.

Hagstrom RM, Billings FT, Chapnick EM et al. Sudden death in survivors of myocardial infarction. Circulation 1964; 29-30 (Suppl 3):91.

Hamer A, Vohra J, Hunt D et al. Prediction of sudden death by electrophysiologic studies in high risk patients surviving acute myocardial infarction. Am J Cardiol 1982; 50:223.

Hammer A. Ein Fall von trombotischen Verschlusse einer der Kranzarterien des Herzens. Wiener Medizinische Wochenschrift 1878; 5:83.

Hammermeister KE, De Rouen TA, Murray JA et al. Effect of aortocoronary saphenous vein bypass grafting on death and sudden death. Comparison of nonrandomized medically and surgically treated cohorts with comparable coronary disease and left ventricular function. Am J Cardiol 1977; 39:925.

Hamperl H. Zur fragmentatio miocardii. Beitr path Anat 1929; 82:597.

Hassler O. The origin of the cell constituting arterial intima thickening. An experimental autoradiographic study with the use of H^3-thymidine. Lab Invest 1970; 2:286.

Hearse DJ, Humphrey SM, Boink ABTJ et al. The calcium paradox: metabolic, electrophysiological, contractile and ultrastructural characteristics in four species. Eur J Cardiol 1978; 7:241.

Heath D. Cardiac fibroma. Br Heart J 1969; 31:656.

Hecht GM, Klues HG, Roberts WC et al. Coexistence of sudden cardiac death and endstage heart failure in familial hypertrophic cardiomyopathy. J Am Coll Cardiol 1993; 22:489.

Helfant RH, Kemp HG, Gorlin R. The interrelation between extent of coronary artery disease, presence of collaterals, ventriculographic abnormalities and hemodynamics. Am J Cardiol 1970; 25:102.

Hellstrom HR. The injury-spasm (ischemia-induced hemostatic vasoconstrictive) and vascular autoregolatory hypothesis of ischemic disease. Resistance vessel-spasm hypothesis of ischemic disease. Am J Cardiol 1982; 49:802.

Herdson PM, Sommers HM, Jennings RB. A comparative study of the fine structure of normal and ischemic dog myocardium with special reference to early change following temporary occlusion of a coronary artery. Am J Pathol 1975; 46:367.

Hermans WRM, Rensing BJ, Foley DP et al. Therapeutic dissection after successful coronary balloon angioplasty: no influence on restenosis or on clinical outcome in 693 patients. J Am Coll Cardiol 1992; 20:767.

Herrick JB. Clinical features of sudden obstruction of the coronary arteries. JAMA 1912; 59:87.

Herrick JB. Thrombosis of the coronary arteries. JAMA 1919; 72:93.

Hess ML, Hastillo A, Mohanakumar T et al. Accelerated atherosclerosis in cardiac transplantation: role of cytotoic B-cell antibodies and hyperlipidemia. Circulation 1983; 68 (3 part 2):II94.

Hinkle LE, Argyros DC, Hayes JC et al. Pathogenesis of an unexpected sudden death: role of early cycle ventricular premature contractions. Am J Cardiol 1977; 39:873.

Hirai T, Fujita M, Nakajima H et al. Importance of collateral circulation for prevention of left ventricular aneurysm formation in acute myocardial infarction. Circulation 1989; 79:791.

Hombach V, Höher M, Kochs M et al. Pathophysiology of unstable angina pectoris-correlations with coronary angioscopic imaging. Eur Heart J 1988;(Suppl N):40.

Hood WB. Experimental myocardial infarction III Recovery of left ventricular function in the healing phase. Contribution of increased fiber shortening in noninfarcted myocardium. Am Heart J 1970; 79:531.

Hori M, Gotoh K, Kitakaze M et al. Role of oxygen-derived free radicals in myocardial edema and ischemia in coronary microvascular embolization. Circulation 1991; 84:828.

Hort W. Mikroskopische Beobachtung an menschlichen Infarktherzen. Virchow Arch Path Anat 1968; 345:61.

Hottenrott C, Buckerg GD. Studies of the effects of ventricular fibrillation on the adequacy of regional myocardial flow. Electrical versus spontaneous fibrillation. J Thorac Cardiovasc Surg 1974; 68:615.

Hunt D, Gore I. Myocardial lesion following experimental intracranial hemorrhage: prevention with propranolol. Am Heart J 1972; 83:232.

Hurst JW. Notes on teaching: how some words prevent teaching. JAMA 1967; 74:858.

Hutchins GM, Bulkley BH, Ridolfi RL et al. Correlation of coronary arteriograms and left ventriculograms with postmortem studies. Circulation 1977; 56:32.

Huttner I, More RH, Rona G. Fine structural evidence of specific mechanism for increased endothelial permeability in experimental hypertension. Am J Path 1970; 61:395.

Ideker RE, Behar VS, Wagner GS et al. Evaluation of asynergy as an indicator of myocardial fibrosis. Circulation 1978; 57:715.

Irniger W. Histologische Alterbestimmung von Thrombosen und Embolien. Virch Arch path Anat 1963; 336:220.

Jacoby RM, Nesto RW. Acute myocardial infarction in the diabetic patient: pathophysiology, clinical course and prognosis. J Am Coll Cardiol 1992; 20:736.

James TN. Pathology of small coronary arteries. Am J Cardiol 1967; 20:679.

James TN. De Subitaneis Mortibus. VIII. Coronary arteries and conduction system in scleroderma heart disease. Circulation 1974; 50:844.

James TN. De Subitaneis Mortibus. XIX. On the cause of sudden death in pheochromocytoma, with special reference to the pulmonary arteries, the cardiac conduction system and the aggregation of platelets. Circulation 1976; 54:348.

James TN. De Subitaneis Mortibus. XXIII. Rheumatoid arthritis and ankylosing spondylitis. Circulation 1977a;55:669.

James TN. De Subitaneis Mortibus. XXIV. Ruptured interventricular septum and heart block. Circulation 1977b;55:934.

James TN. De Subitaneis Mortibus. XXV. Sarcoid heart disease. Circulation 1977c;56:320.

James TN. De Subitaneis Mortibus. XXVIII. Apoplexy of the heart. Circulation 1978; 57:385.

James TN. Morphologic substrates of sudden death: summary. J Am Coll Cardiol 1985; 5:81B.

James TN. Degenerative lesions of a coronary chemoreceptor and nearby neural elements in the heart of victims of sudden death. J Am Coll Cardiol 1986; 8:12A.

James TN, Armstrong RS, Silverman J et al. De Subitaneis Mortibus. VI. Two young soldiers. Circulation 1974; 49:1239.

James TN, Beeson CW II, Sherman EB et al. De Subitaneis Mortibus. XIII. Multifocal Purkinje cell tumors of the heart. Circulation 1975; 52:333.

James TN, Carson NAJ, Froggatt P. De Subitaneis Mortibus. IV. Coronary vessels and conduction system in homocystinuria. Circulation 1974; 49:367.

James TN, Derek JL, Carson DJ et al. De Subitaneis Mortibus.1. Fibroma compressing His bundle. Circulation 1973a;48:428.

James TN, Frame B, Coates EO. De Subitaneis Mortibus. III. Pickwickian syndrome. Circulation 1973c;48:1311.

James TN, Froggatt P, Atkinsons WJ Jr et al. De Subitaneis Mortibus. XXX. Observations on the pathophysiology of the long QT syndromes with special reference to the neuropathology of the heart. Circulation 1978; 57:1221.

James TN, Froggatt P, Marshall TK. De Subitaneis Mortibus. II. Coronary embolism in the fetus. Circulation 1973b;48:890.

James TN, Galakhov I. De Subitaneis Mortibus. XXVI. Fatal electrical instability of the heart associated with benign congenital polycystic tumor of the atrioventricular node. Circulation 1977; 56:667.

James TN, Hackel DB, Marshall TK. De Subitaneis Mortibus. V. Occluded A-V node artery. Circulation 1974; 49:772.

James TN, Haubrich WS. De Subitaneis Mortibus. XIV. Bacterial arteritis in Whipple's disease. Circulation 1975; 52:722.

James TN, Jackson DA. De Subitaneis Mortibus. XXVII. Histological abnormalities in the sinus node, atrioventricular node and His bundle associated with coarctation of the aorta. Circulation 1977; 56:1094.

James TN, Marilley RJ Ir, Marriott HJ. De Subitaneis Mortibus. XI. Young girl with palpitations. Circulation 1975; 51:743.

James TN, Marshall ML, Craig MW. De Subitaneis Mortibus. VII. Disseminated intravascular coagulation and paroxysmal atrial tachycardia. Circulation 1974; 50:395.

James TN, Marshall TK. De Subitaneis Mortibus. XII. Asymmetrical hypertrophy of the heart. Circulation 1975; 51:1149.

James TN, Marshall TK. De Subitaneis Mortibus. XVII. Multifocal stenoses due to fibromuscular dysplasia of the sinus node artery. Circulation 1976a;53:736.

James TN, Marshall TK. De Subitaneis Mortibus. XVIII. Persistent fetal dispersion of the atrioventricular node and His bundle within the central fibrous body. Circulation 1976b53:1026.

James TN, Marshall TK, Edwards JE. De Subitaneis Mortibus. XX. Cardiac electrical instability in the presence of a left superior vena cava. Circulation 1976; 54:689.

James TN, McKone RC, Hudspeth AS. De Subitaneis Mortibus. X. Familial congenital heart block. Circulation 1975; 51:379.

James TN, Pearce WN, Givhan EG. Sudden death while driving. Role of sinus perinodal degeneration and cardiac neural degeneration and ganglionitis. Am J Cardiol 1980; 45:1095.

James TN, Puech P. De Subitaneis Mortibus. IX. Type A Wolff-Parkinson-White Syndrome. Circulation 1974; 50:1264.

James TN, Robertson BT, Waldo AL et al. De Subitaneis Mortibus. XV. Hereditary stenosis of the His bundle in pug dogs. Circulation 1975; 52:1152.

James TN, Schlant RC, Marshall TK. De Subitaneis Mortibus. XXIX. Randomly distributed focal myocardial lesions causing destruction in the His bundle or a narrow-origin left bundle branch. Circulation 1978; 57:816.

James TN, Spencer MS, Kloepfer JC. De Subitaneis Mortibus. XXI. Adult onset syncope, with comments on the nature of congenital heart block and the morphogenesis of the human atrioventricular septal junction. Circulation 1976; 54:1001.

Jennings RB. Early phase of myocardial ischemic injury and infarction. Am J Cardiol 1969; 24:753.

Johnson DW, Flemma RJ, Lepley D. Direct reconstruction of flow to small distal coronary arteries. Am J Cardiol 1970; 25:105.

Jones CE, Devous MD, Thomas JX et al. The effect of chronic cardiac denervation on infarct size following acute coronary occlusion. Am Heart J 1978; 95:738.

Jorgensen L, Haerem JW, Chandler BA et al. The pathology of acute coronary death. Acta Anesth Scand 1968; 29:193.

Jorgensen L, Hovig T, Rowsell HC et al. Adenosine-diphosphate-induced platelet aggregation and vascular injury in swine and rabbits. Am J Path 1970; 61:161.

Jorgensen L, Rowsell HC, Hovig T et al. Adenosine-diphosphate-induced platelet aggregation and myocardial infarction in swine. Lab Invest 1967; 17:616.

Jost S, Deckers JW, Nikutta P et al. Progression of coronary artery disease is dependent on anatomic location and diameter. J Am Coll Cardiol 1993; 2:1339.

Kahn JP, Perumal AS, Gully RJ et al. Correlation of type A behaviour with adrenergic receptor density: implications for coronary artery disease pathogenesis. Lancet 1987; 24:937.

Kannel WB, Doyle JT, McNamara P et al. Precursors of sudden coronary death. Factors related to the incidence of sudden death. Circulation 1975; 51:606.

Kannel WB, Schatzkin A. Sudden death: lessons from subsets in population studies. J Am Coll Cardiol 1985; 5:141B.

Kaplan J. The influence of sympathetic activation and psychosocial stress on coronary artery atherosclerosis. In Hypertension -The tip of an iceberg; In Therapeutics Today Series. Manchester: Adis Press, 1988;l7:9.

Kaplan JR, Manuck SB, Adams MR et al. The effects of beta-adrenergic blocking agents on atherosclerosis and its complications. Eur Heart J 1987; 8:928.

Kassab GS, Imoto K, White FC et al. Coronary arterial tree remodeling in right ventricular hypertrophy. Am J Physiol 1993; 265(Heart Circ Physiol 34): H366.

Katz AM. Effects of ischemia on the cardiac contractile proteins. Cardiology 1971-72; 56:276.

Katz AM. Cellular mechanisms in congestive heart failure. Am J Cardiol 1988; 62:3A.

Kaunitz PE. Origin of left coronary artery from pulmonary artery. Review of the literature and report of two cases. Am Heart J 1947; 33:182.

Kern WH, Dermer GB, Lindesmith GG. The intimal proliferation in aortic-coronary saphenous vein grafts. Light and electron microscopic studies. Am Heart J 1972; 84:771.

Khouri EM, Gregg DE, Lowesohn HS. Flow in the major branches of the left coronary artery during experimental coronary insufficiency in the unanesthetized dog. Circ Res 1968; 23:99.

Khouri EM, Gregg DE, McGranahan GM. Regression and reappearance of coronary collaterals. Am J Physiol 1971; 220:655.

Kloner RA, Allen J, Zheng Y et al. Myocardial stunning following exercise treadmill testing in man. J Am Coll Cardiol 1990; 15:203A.

Kloner RA, Ganote CE, Jennings RB. The "no-reflow" phenomenon after temporary coronary occlusion in the dog. J Clin Invest 1974; 54:1496.

Kloner RA, Przyklenk K, Patel B. Altered myocardial states. The stunned and hibernating myocardium. Am J Med 1989; 86 (Supp 1A):14.

Knisely MH. The settling of sludge during life. First observations, evidences and significance. A contribution to the biophysics of disease. Acta Anat 1961; 44:7.

Kochi K, Takebayashi S, Hikori T et al. Significance of adventitial inflammation of the coronary artery in patients with unstable angina: Results at autopsy. Circulation 1985; 71:709.

Kosek JC, Chartrand C, Hurley EJ et al. Arteries in canine cardiac homografts. Ultrastructure during acute rejection. Lab Invest 1969; 21:328.

Kragel AH, Gertz SD, Roberts WC. Morphologic comparison of frequency and types of acute lesions in the major epicardial coronary arteries in unstable angina pectoris, sudden coronary death and acute myocardial infarction. J Am Coll Cardiol 1991; 18:801.

Kragel AH, Reddy SG, Wittes JT et al. Morphometric analysis of the composition of atherosclerotic plaques in the four major epicardial coronary arteries in acute myocardial infarction and sudden coronary death. Circulation 1989; 80:1747.

Kubler W. The sympathetic system in evolution and in ischemic heart disease: a controversy? Eur Heart J 1992; 13:1301.

Kubler W, Strasser RH. Signal transduction in myocardial ischemia. Eur Heart J 1994; 15:437.

Kuller L, Perper J, Cooper M. Demographic characteristics and trends in arteriosclerotic heart disease mortality: sudden death and myocardial infarction. Circulation 1975; 51/52 (suppl.3):1.

La Canna G, Alfieri O, Giubbini R et al. Echocardiography during infusion of dobutamine for identification of reversible dysfunction in patients with chronic coronary artery disease. J Am Coll Cardiol 1994; 23:617.

Laks H, Kaiser GC, Mudd JG et al. Revascularization of the right coronary artery. Am J Cardiol 1979; 43:1109.

Lancisi GM. Opera Omnia, Tomus I De Subitaneis Mortibus, Libri duo, Tertia editione, Roma: Palladis, 1970:1745. (Translated by PD White and AV Boursey, St. John's University Press, New York.)

Langille LB. Hemodynamic factors and vascular disease. In: Silver MD ed. Cardiovascular Pathology. 2nd ed. New York: Churchill Livingstone Inc,1991:131.

Leary T. Coronary spasm as a possible factor in producing sudden death. Am Heart J 1935; 10:338.

Lee D, Eigler N, Fishbein MC et al. Identification of intracoronary thrombus and demonstration of thrombectomy by intravascular ultrasound imaging. Am J Cardiol 1994; 73:522.

Lesch M, Kehoe RF. Predictability of sudden cardiac death: a partially fulfilled promise. N Engl J Med 1984; 310:255.

Lev M, Watne AL. Method for routine histopathologic study of human sinoatrial node. Arch Path 1954; 57:168.

Lev M, Widran J, Erickson EE. A method for histopathological study of A-V node bundle and branches. Arch Path 1951; 52:73.

Levin DC, Fallon JT. Significance of the angiographic morphology of localized coronary stenoses: histopathologic correlations. Circulation 1982; 66:316.

Levine HD, Welles RE. Blood sludging observed at the bedside: flexibility and limitations of examination by ophthalmoscopy. Am J Cardiol 1964; 13:48.

Levy RL, Breunn HG. Acute coronary insufficiency. JAMA 1936; 106:1080.

Liberthson RR, Nagel EL, Hirschman JC et al. Pathophysiologic observations in prehospital ventricular fibrillation and sudden cardiac death. Circulation 1974; 49:790.

Lie JT. Histopathology of the conduction system in sudden death from coronary heart disease. Circulation 1975; 51:446.

Lie JT. Sudden death from diseases of the cardiovascular system. In: Silver MD, ed. Cardiovascular Pathology. 2nd ed. New York: Churchill Livingstone Inc, 1991:811.

Lie JT, Lawrie GM, Morris GC et al. Hemorrhagic myocardial infarction associated with aortocoronary bypass revascularization. Am Heart J 1978; 96:295.

Lie JT, Titus JL. Pathology of the myocardium and the conduction system in sudden coronary death. Circulation 1975; 51-52(Suppl 3):41.

Likar IN, Robinson RW, Gouvelis A. Microthrombi and intimal thickening in bovine coronary arteries. Arch Path 1969; 87:146.

Linzbach AJ. Mikrometrische und histologische Analyse hypertropher menschlicher Herzen. Virchows Arch Path Anat 1947; 314:534.

Lisa JR. Pathologic findings in the heart in sudden cardiac deaths. Ann Intern Med 1939; 12:1968.

Little WC, Constantinescu M, Applegate RJ et al. Can coronary angiography predict the site of a subsequent myocardial infarction in patients with mild-to-moderate coronary artery disease? Circulation 1988; 78:1157.

Liuzzo G, Biasucci ML, Gallimore RJ et al. The prognostic value of C-reactive protein and serum amyloid A protein in severe unstable angina. N Engl J Med 1994; 331:417.

Lowe JE, Cummings RG, Adams DH et al. Evidence that ischemic cell death begins in the subendocardium independent of variations in collateral flow or wall tension. Circulation 1983; 68:190.

Lown B. Sudden cardiac death: the major challenge confronting contemporary cardiology. Am J Cardiol 1979; 43:313.

Lown B, Verrier RL, Rabinowitz SH. Neural and psychologic mechanisms and the problem of sudden cardiac death. Am J Cardiol 1977; 39:890.

Ludwig G. Capillary pattern of the myocardium. In: Bajusz E, Jasmin G, eds. Functional Morphology of the Heart. Basel: Karger, Meth Achievm Exp Path,5.1971:238.

Luke JL, Helpern M. Sudden unexpected death from natural causes in young adults. A review of 275 consecutive autopsied cases. Arch Path 1968; 85:10.

Lum M, Stevenson WG, Stevenson LW et al. Diverse mechanisms of unexpected cardiac arrest in advanced heart failure. Circulation 1989; 80:1675.

Lynch JJ, Paskewitz DA, Gimbel KS et al. Psychological aspects of cardiac arrhythmia. Am Heart J 1977; 93:645.

MacIsaac AI, Thomas JD, Topol EJ. Toward the quiescent coronary plaque. J Am Coll Cardiol 1993; 22:1228.

Maisel AS. Beneficial effects of metaprolol treatment in congestive heart failure. Reversal of sympathetic-induced alterations of immunologic function. Circulation 1994; 90:1774.

Majno G, Ames A, Chaing J et al. No-reflow after cerebral ischemia. Lancet 1967; 2:569.

Mak T, Weiglicki WB. Protection by beta-blocking agents against free radical-mediated sarcolemmal lipid peroxidation. Circ Res 1988; 63:262.

Malliani A, Schwartz PJ, Zanchetti A. A sympathetic reflex elicited by experimental coronary occlusion. Am J Physiol 1979; 217:703.

Mallory GK, White PD, Salcedo-Salgar J. The speed of healing of myocardial infarction. A study of the pathologic anatomy of seventy-two cases. Am Heart J 1939; 18:647.

Mantini E, Tanaka S, Lillehei CW. Analysis of the earliest effects of mammary artery implantation on the ischemic ventricle. Ann Thorac Surg 1968; 5:393.

Manyari DE, Knudtson M, Kloiber R et al. Sequential Thallium-201 myocardial perfusion studies after successful percutaneous transluminal coronary artery angioplasty: delayed resolution of exercise-induced scintigraphic abnormalities. Circulation 1988; 77:86.

Marcus FI, Fontaine GH, Guiraudon G et al. Right ventricular dysplasia: a report of 24 adult cases. Circulation 1982; 65:384.

Marcus ML, Chilian WM, Kanatsuga H et al. Understanding the coronary circulation through studies at the microvascular level. Circulation 1990; 82:1.

Margolis JR, Hirshfeld JW, McNeer FJ et al. Sudden death due to coronary artery disease. A clinical, hemodynamic and angiographic profile. Circulation 1975; 51-52(Suppl 3):180.

Marino P, Nidasio G, Golia G et al. Frequency of predischarge ventricular arrhythmias in postmyocardial infarction patients depends on residual left ventricular pump performance and is independent of the occurrence of acute reperfusion. J Am Coll Cardiol 1994; 23:290.

Maron BJ, Roberts WC, Edwards JE et al. Sudden death in patients with hypertrophic cardiomyopathy: characterization of 26 patients without functional limitation. Am J Cardiol 1978; 41:803.

Maron BJ, Roberts WC, McAllister HA et al. Sudden death in young athletes. Circulation 1980; 62:218.

Marsch SCU, Wanigasekera VA, Ryder WA et al. Graded myocardial ischemia is associated with a decrease in diastolic distensibility of the remote nonischemic myocardium in the anesthetized dog. J Am Coll Cardiol 1993; 22:899.

Marti MC, Bouchardy B, Cox JN. Aortocoronary bypass with autogenous saphenous vein grafts: histopathological aspects. Virchow Arch Path Anat 1971; 152:255.

Martin AM, Hackel DB. The myocardium of the dog in hemorrhagic shock. An histochemical study. Lab Invest 1963; 12:77.

Martin AM, Hackel DB. An electron microscopic study of the progression of myocardial lesions in the dog after hemorrhagic shock. Lab Invest 1966; 15:243.

Maseri A, Crea F, Cianflone D. Myocardial ischemia caused by distal coronary vasoconstriction. Am J Cardiol 1992; 70:1602.

Maseri A, L'Abbate A, Baroldi G et al. Coronary vasospasm as a possible cause of myocardial infarction. A conclusion derived from the study of "pre-infarction" angina. N Engl J Med 1978; 299:1271.

Mathey DG, Kuck KH, Tilsner V et al. Non surgical coronary artery recanalization in acute transmural mycocardial infarction. Circulation 1981; 63:489.

Mazzone A, De Servi S, Ricevuti G et al. Increased expression of neutrophil and monocyte adhesion molecules in unstable coronary artery disease. Circulation 1993; 88:358.

McCance AJ, Thompson PA, Forfar JC. Increased cardiac sympathetic nervous activity in patients with unstable coronary heart disease. Eur Heart J 1993; 14:751.

McFalls EO, Araujo LI, Lammertsma A et al. Vasodilator reserve in collateral-dependent myocardium as measured by positron emission tomography. Eur Heart J 1993; 14:336.

McGill HC, Eggen DA, Guzman MA et al. The geographic pathology of atherosclerosis. Lab Invest 1968; 18:463.

McIntosh HD. Sudden cardiac death. Neural control of the heart: summary of discussion. J Am Coll Cardiol 1985; 5:111B.

Meerson FZ. The myocardium in hyperfunction, hypertophy and heart failure. Circul Res 1969; 25(Suppl 2):1.

Meerson FZ, Kagan VE, Kozlov YP et al. The role of lipid peroxidation in pathogenesis of ischemic damage and the antioxidant protection of the heart. Basic Res Cardiol 1982; 77:465.

Mehmet CO, Roberts CS, Lemole GM. Role of lymphostasis in accelerated atherosclerosis in transplanted heart. Am J Cardiol 1987; 60:430.

Milstein S, Buetikofer J, Lesser J et al. Cardiac asystole: a manifestation of neurally mediated hypotension-bradycardia. J Am Coll Cardiol 1989; 14:1626.

Minkowski WL. The coronary arteries of infants. Am J M Sc 1947; 214:623.

Mitrani RD, Klein LS, Miles WH et al. Regional cardiac sympathetic denervation in patients with ventricular tachycardia in absence of coronary artery disease. J Am Coll Cardiol 1993; 22:1344.

Moberg A. Anastomoses between extracardiac vessels and coronary arteries. Acta Med Scand 1968; 485 (Suppl):1.

Moon HD Coronary arteries in fetuses, infants and juveniles. Circulation 1957; 16:263.

Moore CA, Cannon J, Watson DD et al. Thallium-201 kinetics in stunned myocardium characterized by severe postischemic systolic dysfunction. Circulation 1990; 81:1622.

Morales AR, Romanelli R, Boucek RJ. The mural left anterior descending coronary artery, strenuous exercise and sudden death. Circulation 1980; 62:230.

Morales AR, Romanelli R, Tate LG et al. Intramural left anterior descending coronary artery: significance of the depth of the muscular tunnel. Hum Pathol 1993; 24:693.

Moreno PR, Falk E, Palacios IF et al. Macrophage infiltration in acute coronary syndromes. Implications for plaque rupture. Circulation 1994; 90:775.

Morgagni JB. De Sedibus et Causis Morborum per Anatomen Indagatis. Ebrodani in Elvetia, 1779.

Morgan AD. The Pathogenesis of Coronary Occlusion. Oxford: Blackwell Scientific Publications, 1956.

Moritz AR, Zamcheck N. Sudden and unexpected death of young soldiers: diseases responsible for such death during world war II. Arch Path 1946; 42:459.

Morris JN, Gardner MJ. Epidemiology of ischemic heart disease; Am J Med 1969; 46:674.

Moschos CB, Haider B, Khan Y et al. Relation of platelets to catecholamine induced myocardial injury. Cardiov Res 1978; 12:243.

Munck W. The pathological anatomy of sudden heart death. Acta Path et Microbiol Scandinav 1946; 23:107.

Mustard JF, Packham MA. Platelet function and myocardial infarction. Circulation 1969; 40 (Suppl 4):20.

Myasnikov AL, Chazov EI, Hoshevnikova TL et al. Some new data on the occurrence of coronary thrombosis in conjuction with atherosclerosis. J Atheroscl Res 1961; 1:401.

Nasser FN, Walls JT, Edwards WD et al. Lidocaine-induced reduction in size of experimental myocardial infarction. Am J Cardiol 1980; 46:967.

Nathanson MH. Pathology and pharmacology of cardiac syncope and sudden death. Arch Intern Med 1936; 58:685.

Neri Serneri GG, Abbate R, Gori AM et al. Transient intermittent lymphocyte activation is responsible for the instability of angina. Circulation 1992; 86:790.

Neri Serneri GG, Boddi M, Arata L et al. Silent ischemia in unstable angina is related to an altered cardiac norepinephrine handling. Circulation 1993; 87:1928.

Nesto R, Kowalchuk G. The ischemic cascade: temporal sequence of hemodynamic, electrocardiographic and symptomatic expression of ischemia. Am J Cardiol 1987; 59:23C.

Newman WP, Tracy RE, Strong JP et al. Pathology of sudden coronary death. Ann NY Acad Sci 1982; 382:39.

Noakes TD, LH Opie. Marathon running and the heart: the South African experience. Am Heart J 1979a;98:669.

Noakes TD, LH Opie, Rose AG. Autopsy-proved coronary atherosclerosis in marathon runners. N Engl J Med 1979b;301:86.

Noble J, Bourassa MG, Peticlerc R et al. Myocardial bridging and milking effect of the left anterior descending coronary artery: normal variant or obstruction? Am J Cardiol 1976; 37:993.

Nohara R, Kambara H, Murakami T et al. Collateral function in early acute myocardial infarction. Am J Cardiol 1983; 52:955.

O'Reilly RJ, Spellberg RD. Rapid resolution of coronary arterial emboli. Myocardial infarction and subsequent normal coronary arteriograms. Ann Intern Med 1974; 81:348.

Oka M, Angrist A. Histoenzymatic studies of vessels in hypertensive rats. Lab Invest 1967; 16:25.

Oliva PB, Breckinridge JC. Arteriographic evidence of coronary arterial spasm in acute myocardial infarction. Circulation 1977; 56:366.

Oliva PB, Hammill SC, Edwards WD. Cardiac rupture, a clinically predictable complication of acute myocardial infarction: report of 70 cases with clinicopathologic correlations. J Am Coll Cardiol 1993; 22:720.

Oliva PB, Potts DE, Plus RG. Coronary arterial spasm in Prinzmetal angina. N Engl J Med 1973; 288:745.

Oliver MF. Sudden cardiac death: lessons from epidemiology: summary of general discussion. J Am Coll Cardiol 1985; 5:155B.

Oparil S. Morphologic substrates of sudden death: pathogenesis of ventricular hypertrophy. J Am Coll Cardiol 1985; 5:57B.

Opie L. Sudden death and sport. Lancet 1975; 1:263.

Opie LH. The mechanism of myocyte death in ischaemia. Eur Heart J 1993; 14 (Suppl G):31.

Osborn GR. The incubation period of coronary thrombosis. London: Butterworths, 1963

Packer M. Sudden unexpected death in patients with congestive heart failure: a second frontier. Circulation 1985; 72:681.

Pagenstecher. Weiterer Beitrag zur Herzchirurgie. Die Unterbindung der verletzen Arteria Coronaria. Dtsch Med Wochenschr 1901; 4:56.

Parmley LF, Mattingly TW, Manion WC. Penetrating wounds of the heart and aorta. Circulation 1958; 17:953.

Parmley WW. Factors causing arrhythmias in chronic congestive heart failure. Am Heart J 1987; 114:1267.

Parodi O, De Maria R, Oltrona L et al. Myocardial blood flow distribution in patients with ischemic heart disease or dilated cardiomyopathy undergoing heart transplantation. Circulation 1993; 88:509.

Parums D, Mitchinson MJ. Demonstration of immunoglobulin in the neighbourhood of advanced atherosclerotic plaques. Atherosclerosis 1981; 38:211.

Pasternac A, Tubau JF, Puddu PE et al. Increased plasma catecholamine levels in patients with symptomatic mitral valve prolapse. Am J Med 1982; 73:783.

Paterson JC. Capillary rupture with intimal hemorrhage as a causative factor in coronary thrombosis. Arch Path 1938; 25:474.

Patterson E, Holland K, Eller BT et al. Ventricular fibrillation resulting from ischemia at a site remote from previous myocardial infarction. A conscious canine model of sudden coronary death. Am J Cardiol 1982; 50:1414.

Perper JA, Kuller LH, Cooper M. Arteriosclerosis of coronary arteries in sudden unexpected deaths. Circulation 1975; 51-52(Suppl 3):27.

Peters RW, Mitchell LB, Brooks MM et al. Circadian pattern of arrhythmic death in patients receiving encainide, flecainide or moricizine in the cardiac arrhythmia suppression trial (CAST). J Am Coll Cardiol 1994; 23:283.

Pierard LA, De Landsheere CM, Berthe C et al. Identification of viable myocardium by echocardiography during dobutamine infusion in patients with myocardial infarction after thrombolytic therapy: comparison with positron emission tomography. J Am Coll Cardiol 1990; 15:1021.

Pool J, Kunst K, Wermeskerken van JL. Two monitored cases of sudden death outside hospital. Brit Heart J 1978; 40:627.

Pratt CM, Francis MJ, Luck JC et al. Analysis of ambulatory electrocardiograms in 15 patients during spontaneous ventricular fibrillation with special reference to preceding arrhythmic events. J Am Coll Cardiol 1983; 2:789.

Proust F, Pujet JCP, Lubin S et al. Mort subite au cours d'un enregistrement electrocardiographique continu par la methode de Holter. Arch Mal Coeur 1981; 74:99.

Przyklenk K, Bauer B, Ovize M et al. Regional ischemic 'preconditioning' protects remote virgin myocardium from subsequent sustained coronary occlusion. Circulation 1993; 87:893.

Przyklenk K, Kloner RA. Superoxide dismutase plus catalase improve contractile function in the canine model of the stunned myocardium. Circ Res 1986; 58:148.

Pupita G, Maseri A, Kaski J C et al. Myocardial ischemia caused by distal coronary-artery constriction in stable angina pectoris. N Engl J Med 1990; 323:514.

Quyyumi AA, Diodati JG, Lakatos E et al. Angiogenic effects of low molecular weight heparin in patients with stable coronary artery disease: a pilot study. J Am Coll Cardiol 1993; 22:635.

Raab W. Preventive Myocardiology, Fundamentals and Targets. In: Kugelmass NI, (ed), Bannerstone Division of American Lectures in Living Chemistry. Springfield,III: CC Thomas, 1970

Rabson MS, Helpern M. Sudden and unexpected death. II Coronary atherosclerosis. Am Heart J 1948; 35:63.

Rafflenbeul W, Smith LR, Rogers WL et al. Quantitative coronary arteriography. Coronary anatomy of patients with unstable angina pectoris reexamined 1 year after optimal medical therapy. Am J Cardiol 1979; 43:699.

Rahimtoola SH. The hibernating myocardium. Am Heart J 1989; 117:21.

Reduto LA, Freund GC, Gaeta JM et al. Coronary artery reperfusion in acute myocardial infarction: beneficial effects of intracoronary streptokinase on left ventricula salvage and performance. Am Heart J 1981; 102:1168.

Reichenbach DD, Benditt EP. Myofibrillar degeneration: a common form of cardiac muscle injury. Ann NY Ac Sci 1969; 156:164.

Reichenbach DD, Benditt EP. Catecholamine and cardiomiopathy: the pathogenesis and potential importance of myofibrillar degeneration. Hum Path 1970; 1:125.

Reichenbach DD, Moss NS. Myocardial cell necrosis and sudden death in humans. Circulation 1975; 51-52(Suppl 3):60.

Reichenbach DD, Moss NS, Meyer E. Pathology of the heart in sudden cardiac death. Am J Cardiol 1977; 39:865.

Reimer KA, Jennings RB. The changing anatomic reference base of evolving myocardial infarction. Understimation of myocardial collateral blood flow and overestimation of experimental anatomic infarct size due to edema, hemorrhage and acute inflammation. Circulation 1979; 60:866.

Reimer KA, Lowe JE, Rasmussen MM et al. The wavefront phenomenon of ischemic cell death. I Myocardial infarct size vs duration of coronary occlusion in dogs. Circulation 1977; 56:786.

Reimer KA, Rasmussen MM, Jennings RB. On the nature of protection by propranolol against myocardial necrosis after temporary coronary occlusion in dogs. Am J Cardiol 1976; 37:520.

Rentrop KP, Cohen M, Blanke H et al. Changes in collateral channel filling immediately after controlled coronary artery occlusion by an angioplasty balloon in human subjects. J Am Coll Cardiol 1985; 5:587.

Rentrop KP, Feit F, Sherman W et al. Late thrombolytic therapy preserves left ventricular function in patients with collateralized total coronary occlusion: primary end point findings of the second Mount Sinai-New York University reperfusion trial. J Am Coll Cardiol 1989a;14:58.

Rentrop KP, Feit F, Sherman W et al. Serial angiographic assessment of coronary artery obstruction and collateral flow in acute myocardial infarction. Report from the second Mount Sinai-New Yok University reperfusion trial. Circulation 1989b;80:1166.

Rentrop KP, Thornton JC, Feit F et al. Determinants and protective potential of coronary arterial collaterals as assessed by an angioplasty model. Am J Cardiol 1988; 61:67.

Rider AK, Bieber PP, Harrison DC. Atherosclerosis in long-term survivors of human cardiac allograft transplantation. Circulation 1972; 46 (Suppl 2):77.

Ridolfi RL, Hutchins GM. The relationship between coronary artery lesions and myocardial infarcts: ulceration of atherosclerotic plaques precipitating coronary thrombosis. Am Heart J 1977; 93:468.

Rigo P, Becker LC, Griffith LSC et al. Influence of coronary collateral vessels on the results of thallium-201 myocardial stress imaging. Am J Cardiol 1979; 44:452.

Roberts WC, Buja LM. The frequency and significance of coronary arterial thrombi and other observations in fatal acute myocardial infarction. Am J Med 1972; 52:425.

Roberts WC, Curry RC, Isner JM et al. Sudden death in Prinzmetal's angina with coronary spasm documented by angiography. Analysis of three necropsy patients. Am J Cardiol 1982; 50:203.

Roberts WC, Jones AA. Quantitation of coronary arterial narrowing at necropsy in sudden coronary death. Analysis of 31 patients and comparison with 25 control subjects. Am J Cardiol 1979; 44:39.

Roberts WC, Siegel RJ, Zipes DP. Origin of the right coronary artery from the left sinus of Valsalva and its functional consequences: analysis of 10 necropsy patients. Am J Cardiol 1982; 49:863-868.

Rodbard S. Vascular modifications induced by flow. Am Heart J 1956; 51:926.

Rodbard S. Physical factors in arterial sclerosis and stenosis. Angiology 1971; 22:267.

Rogers WJ, Hood WP, Mantle JA et al. Return of left ventricular function after reperfusion in patients with myocardial infarction: importance of sub-total stenoses or intact collaterals. Circulation 1984; 69:338.

Rona G, Chappel CI, Balazs T et al. An infarct-like myocardial lesion and other toxic manifestations produced by isoproterenol in rat. Arch Path 1959; 67:443.

Rose AG, Uys CJ. Pathology of cardiac transplantation. In: Silver MD, ed. Cardiovascular Pathology. 2nd ed. New York: Churchill Livingstone Inc, 1991:1649.

Rosenschein U, Ellis SG, Haudenschild CC et al. Comparison of histopathologic coronary lesions obtained from directional atheroctomy in stable angina versus acute coronary syndromes. Am J Cardiol 1994; 73:508.

Ross R. The arterial wall and atherosclerosis. Ann Rev Med 1979; 30:1.

Ross R. The pathogenesis of atherosclerosis: a perspective for the 1990s. Nature 1993; 362:801.

Rossi L. Pathologic changes in the cardiac conduction and nerve system in sudden coronary death. Ann NY Acad Sci 1982; 382:50.

Rossi L: Cardioneuropathy and extracardiac neural disease. J Am Coll Cardiol 1985; 5 (Suppl 6):66B.

Rossi L, Matturri L. Clinicopathologic approach to cardiac arrhythmias. A color atlas. Torino: Centro Scientifico Torinese, Italy,1990.

Ruffer MA. On arterial lesions found in Egyptian Mummies. J Path Bact 1911; 15:453.

Sabbah HN, Goldberg AD, Schoels W et al. Spontaneous and inducible ventricular arrhythmias in a canine model of chronic heart failure: relation to haemodynamics and sympathoadrenergic activation. Eur Heart J 1992; 13:1562.

Saber RS, Edwards WD, Bailey KR et al. Coronary embolization after balloon angioplasty or thrombolytic therapy: an autopsy study of 32 cases. J Am Coll Cardiol 1993; 22:1283.

Sabia PJ, Powers ER, Jayaweera AR. Functional significance of collateral blood flow in patients with recent acute myocardial infarction. A study using myocardial contrast echocardiography. Circulation 1992a;85:2080.

Sabia PJ, Powers ER, Ragosta M et al. An association between collateral blood flow and myocardial viability in patients with recent myocardial infarction. N Engl J Med 1992b;327:1825.

Saffitz JE, Sazama K, Roberts WC. Amyloidosis limited to small arteries causing angina pectoris and sudden death. Am J Cardiol 1983; 51:1234.

Saito Y, Yasuno M, Ishida M et al. Importance of coronary collaterals for restoration of left ventricular function after intracoronary thrombolysis. Am J Cardiol 1985; 55:1259.

Saphir O. Anatomical evidence of functional disorders of the heart. Arch Path 1933; 16:315.

Saphir O, Kasner HT. An anatomical and experimental study of segmentation of the myocardium and its relationship to the intercalated disc. J Med Res 1924; 44:539.

Sasaki H, Hoshi H, Hong YM et al. Purification of acidic fibroblast growth factor from bovine heart and its localization in the cardiac myocytes. J Biol Chem 1989; 264:17606.

Sasayama S, Masatoshi F. Recent insights into coronary collateral circulation. Circulation 1992; 85:1197.

Schaper J, Borgers M, Schaper W. Ultrastructure of ischemia-induced changes in the precapillary anastomotic network of the heart. Am J Cardiol 1972; 29:851.

Scheel KW, Seavey E, Gaugl JF et al. Coronary and myocardial adaptations to high altitude in dogs. Am J Physiol 1990; 259 (Heart Circ Physiol 28) H1667.

Scheel KW, Williams SE. Hypertrophy and coronary and collateral vascularity in dogs with severe chronic anemia. Am J Physiol 1985; 249 (Heart Circ Physiol 18) H103.

Schlesinger MJ. Relation of anatomic pattern to pathological conditions of the coronary arteries. Arch Path 1940; 30:403.

Schlesinger MJ, Reiner L. Focal myocytolysis of the heart. Am J Path 1955; 31:443.

Schornagel HE. Intimal thickening in the coronary arteries in infants. Arch Path 1956; 62:427.

Schroder ES, Sirna SJ, Kieso RA et al. Sensitization of reperfused myocardium to subsequent coronary flow reductions. An extension of the concept of myocardial stunning. Circulation 1988; 78:717.

Schwaiger M, Schelbert HR, Ellison D et al. Sustained regional abnormalities in cardiac metabolism after transient ischemia in the chronic dog model. J Am Coll Cardiol 1985; 6:336.

Schwartz CJ, Mitchell JRA. Cellular infiltration of the human arterial adventitia associated with atheromatous plaque. Circulation 1962; 26:73.

Schwartz H, Leiboff RH, Bren GB et al. Temporal evolution of the human coronary collateral circulation after myocardial infarction. J Am Coll Cardiol 1984; 4:1088.

Schwartz H, Leiboff RH, Katz KJ et al. Arteriographic predictors of spontaneous improvement in left ventricular function after myocardial infarction. Circulation 1985; 71:466.

Schwartz PJ, Billman GE, Stone HL. Autonomic mechanisms in ventricular fibrillation induced by myocardial ischemia during exercise in dogs with healed myocardial infarction. Circulation 1984; 69:790.

Schwartz PJ, La Rovere MT, Vanoli E. Autonomic nervous system and sudden cardiac death. Experimental basis and clinical observations for post-myocardial infarction risk stratification. Circulation 1992; 85 (Suppl 1):1-77.

Schwarz F, Schaper J, Becker V et al. Coronary collateral vessels: their significance for left ventricular histologic structure. Am J Cardiol 1982; 49:291.

Scott RF, Briggs TS. Pathologic findings in pre-hospital deaths due to coronary atherosclerosis. Am J Cardiol 1972; 29:782.

Serruys PW, Wijns W, Van den Brand M et al. Left ventricular performance, regional blood flow, wall motion, and lactate metabolism during transluminal angioplasty. Circulation 1984; 70:25.

Sharma B, Asinger R, Francis G et al. Demonstration of exercise-induced painless myocardial ischemia in survivors of out-of-hospital ventricular fibrillation. Am J Cardiol 1987; 59:740.

Shen AC, Jennings RB. Unusual features of cell injury in cells on the edge of myocardial infarcts. Am J Path 1971; 62: abs.171.

Sherman CT, Litvack F, Grundfest WS et al. Demonstration of thrombus and complex atheroma by in-vivo angioscopy in patients with unstable angina pectoris. N Eng J Med 1986; 315:913.

Shvalev VN, Virkhert AM, Stropus RA et al. Changes in neural and humoral mechanisms of the heart in sudden death due to myocardial abnormalities. J Am Coll Cardiol 1986; 8:55A.

Silver MD. Medial hemorrhage and dissection in a coronary artery: an unusual cause of coronary occlusion. CMAJ 1968; 99:32.

Silver MD, Baroldi G, Mariani F. The relationship between acute occlusive coronary thrombi and myocardial infarction studies in 100 consecutive patients. Circulation 1980; 61:219.

Silver MD, Butany J, Chiasson D. The pathology of myocardial infarction and its mechanical complications. In: David TE, ed. Mechanical complications of Myocardial Infarction. Austin TX: Landes, 1993:4.

Silver MD, Wigle ED, Trimble AS et al. Iatrogenic coronary ostial stenosis. Arch Path 1969; 88:73.

Silver MM, Freedom RM. Gross examination and structure of the heart. In: Silver MD, ed. Cardiovascular Pathology, 2nd ed. New York: Churchill Livingston Inc, 1991:1.

Sinusas AJ, Hardin NJ, Clements JP et al. Pathoanatomic correlates of regional left ventricular wall motion assessed by equilibrium radionuclide angiocardiography: a postmortem correlation. Am J Cardiol 1984; 54:975.

Skinner JE. Regulation of cardiac vulnerability by the cerebral defense system. J Am Coll Cardiol 1985; 5:88B.

Smith SH, Kirling JK, Geer JC et al. Arteritis in cardiac rejection after transplantation. Am J Cardiol 1987; 59:1171.

Snow PID, Jones AM, Daber KS. Coronary disease: a pathological study. Brit Heart J 1955; 17:503.

Sommers HM, Jennings RB. Ventricular fibrillation and myocardial necrosis after transient ischemia. Effect of treatment with oxygen, procainamide, reserpine and propranolol. Arch Int Med 1972; 129:780.

Spain DM. Sudden death from coronary artery disese: survival time, frequency of thrombi and cigarette smoking. Am J Cardiol 1970; 25:129.

Spain DM, Bradess VA. Postmortem studies on coronary atherosclerosis in one population group. Dis Chest 1959; 36:397.

Spain DM, Bradess VA, Iral P et al. Intercoronary anastomotic channels and sudden unexpected death from advanced coronary atherosclerosis. Circulation 1963; 27:12.

Spalteholz W. Die Arterien der Herzwand. Anatomische Untersuchungen an Menschen und Tieren. Leipsig; S Hirzel, 1924.

Spalteholz W, Hockrein M. Untersuchungen am Koronarsystem: die anatomische und funktionelle Beschaffenheit der Koronarterienwand. Arch Exp Path u Pharmakol 1931; 163:333.

Speir E, Zhou YF, Lee M et al. Fibroblast growth factors are present in adult cardiac myocytes, in vivo. Biochem Biophys Res Commun 1988; 157:1336.

Spiekerman RE, Brandenburg JT, Achor RWP et al. The spectrum of coronary heart disease in a community of 30,000. A clinicopathologic study. Circulation 1962; 25:57.

Spiro D, Lattes RG, Wiener J. The cellular pathology of experimental hypertension. I. Hyperplastic arteriosclerosis. Am J Path 1965; 47:19.

Spiro D, Spotnitz H, Sonnenblick EH. The relation of cardiac fine structure to function. In: Gould SE, ed. Pathology of the Heart and Blood Vessels. Springfield: Charles C Thomas, 1968:131.

Staemmler M: Hertz. In: Kaufmann E. Lehrbuch der speziellen pathologische Anatomie, Berlin: De Gruyter W, 1961:3.

Stahl LD, Aversano T, Ambrosio G et al. Effect of repeated episodes of drug-induced ventricular dyskinesia on subsequent regional function in the dog: comparison with myocardial stunning produced by repeated coronary occlusions. J Am Coll Cardiol 1987; 9:1339.

Still WJS. The pathogenesis of the intimal thickenings produced by hypertension in large arteries in the rat. Lab Invest 1968; 19:84.

Stinson EB, Billingham ME. Correlative study of regional left ventricular histology and contractile function. Am J Cardiol 1977; 39:378.

Strong JP, Solberg LA, Restrepo C. Atherosclerosis in persons with coronary heart disease. Lab Invest 1968; 18:527.

Summers WK, Jamison RL. The no-reflow phenomenon in renal ischemia. Lab Invest 1971; 25:635.

Sun SC, Burch GE, De Pasquale NP. Histochemical and electron microscopy study of heart muscle after beta-adrenergic blockade. Am Heart J 1967; 74:340.

Surawicz B. Ventricular fibrllation. J Am Coll Cardiol 1985; 5(Suppl6):42B.

Szakacs JE, Cannon A. L-norepinephrine myocarditis. Am J Clin Pathol 1958; 30:425.

Szakacs JE, Dimmette RM, Gowart EC. Pathologic implication of the catecholamines, epinephrine and norepinephrine. U.S. Armed Forces Med J 1959; 10:908.

Taki J, Yasuda T, Gold HK et al. Characteristic of transient left ventricular dysfunction detected by ambulatory left ventricular function monitoring device in patients with coronary artery disease (abstract). Circulation 1987; 76 (Suppl 4):IV 366.

Taylor AL, Murphree S, Buja ML et al. Segmental systolic response to brief ischemia and reperfusion in the hypertrophied canine left ventricle. J Am Coll Cardiol 1992a;20:994.

Taylor AJ, Rogan KM, Virmani R. Sudden cardiac death associated with isolated congenital coronary artery anomalies. J Am Coll Cardiol 1992b;20:640.

Tennant R, Grayzel DM, Sutherland FA et al. Studies on experimental coronary occlusion. Chemical and anatomical changes in the myocardium after coronary ligation. Am Heart J 1936; 12:168.

Tennant R, Wiggers CJ. The effect of the coronary occlusion on myocardial contraction. Am J Physiol 1935; 112:351.

Thiene G, Gambino A, Corrado D et al. The pathological spectrum underlying sudden death in athletes. New Trends in Arrhythmias 1985; 3:323.

Thiene G, Nava A, Corrad D et al. Right ventricular cardiomyopathy and sudden death in young people. N Engl J Med 1988; 318:12.

Thiene G, Pennelli N, Rossi L. Cardiac conduction system abnormalities as a possible cause of sudden death in young athletes. Hum Pathol 1983; 14:709.

Thompson PD, Stern MP, Williams P et al. Death during jogging or running: a study of 18 cases.JAMA 1979; 242:1265.

Thomson JG. Production of severe atheroma in a transplanted human heart. Lancet 1969; 2:1088.

Tillmanns H, Ikeda S, Hansen H et al. Microcirculation in the ventricle of the dog and turtle. Circ Res 1974; 34:561.

Titus JL, Oxman HA, Nobrega FT et al. Sudden unexpected death as the initial manifestation of ischemic heart disease. Clinical and pathologic observations. Am J Cardiol 1970; 26:662.

Todd GL, Baroldi G, Pieper GM et al. Experimental catecholamine-induced myocardial necrosis. I. Morphology, quantification and regional distribution of acute contraction band lesions. J Mol Cell Cardiol 1985a;17:317.

Todd GL, Baroldi G, Pieper GM et al. Experimental catecholamine-induced myocardial necrosis. II Temporal development of isoproterenol-induced contraction band lesions correlated with ECG, hemodynamic and biochemical changes. J Mol Cell Cardiol 1985b;17:647.

Tomoike H, Ross Jr J, Franklin D et al. Improvement by propranolol of regional myocardial dysfunction and abnormal coronary flow pattern in conscious dogs with coronary narrowing. Am J Cardiol 1978; 41:689.

Topol EJ, Ellis SG. Coronary collaterals revisited—accessory pathway to myocardial preservation during infarction. Circulation 1991; 83:1084.

Tsung SH, Huang TY, Chang III. Sudden death in young athletes. Arch Pathol Lab Med 1982; 106:168.

Turitto G, Risa AL, Zanchi E et al. The signal-averaged electrocardiogram and ventricular arrhythmias after thrombolysis for acute myocardial infarction. J Am Coll Cardiol 1990; 15:1270.

Unger EF, Sheffield CD, Epstein SE. Creation of anastomoses between an extracardiac artery and the coronary circulation. Circulation 1990; 82:1449.

Uren NG, Marracini P, Gistri R et al. Altered coronary vasodilator reserve and metabolism in myocardium subtended by normal arteries in patients with coronary artery disease. J Am Coll Cardiol 1993; 22:650.

Uretsky BF, Murali S, Reddy PS et al. Development of coronary artery disease in cardiac transplant patients receiving immuosuppressive therapy with cyclosporine and prednisone. Circulation 1987; 76:827.

Val-Mejias J, Lee WK, Weisse AB et al. Left ventricular performance during and after sickle cell crisis. Am Heart J 1974; 97:585.

Vanderwer MA, Humphrey SM, Gavin JB et al. Changes in the contractile state: fine structure and metabolism of cardiac muscle cells during the development of rigor mortis. Virchows Arch (Cell Pathol) 1981; 35:159.

Vanoverschelde J, Wijns W, Depré C et al. Mechanisms of chronic regional postischemic dysfunction in humans. New insights from the study of noninfarcted collateral-dependent myocardium. Circulation 1993; 87:1513.

Vassable M. On the mechanism underlying cardiac standstill: factors determining success or failure of escape pacemakers in the heart. J Am Coll Cardiol 1985; 5(Suppl6):35B.

Velican C, Velican D. Natural history of coronary atherosclerosis. Boca Raton, Florida: CRC Press Inc, 1989/

Vincent MG, Anderson JL, Marshall HW. Coronary spasm producing coronary thrombosis and myocardial infarction. N Engl J Med 1983; 309:220.

Virmani N, Atkinson JB, Forman MB. Aortocoronary bypass grafts and extracardiac conduits. In: Silver MD, ed. Cardiovascular Pathology. 2nd ed. New York: Churchill Livingstone Inc, 1991:1607.

Virmani R, Robinowitz M, Clark MA et al. Sudden death and partial absence of the right ventricular myocardium. Arch Pathol Lab Med 1982a;106:163.

Virmani R, Robinowitz M, McAllister HA Jr. Nontraumatic death in joggers: a series of 30 patients at autopsy. Am J Med 1982b;72:874.

Vismara LA, Miller RR, Price JE et al. Improved longevity due to reduction of sudden death by aortocoronary bypass in coronary atherosclerosis. Prospective evaluation of medical versus surgical therapy in matched patients with multivessel disease. Am J Cardiol 1977; 39:919.

Vita JA, Treasure CB, Ganz P et al. Control of shear stress in the epicardial coronary arteries of humans: impairment by atherosclerosis. J Am Coll Cardiol 1989; 14:1193.

Vlay SC, Burger L, Vlay LC et al. Prediction of sudden cardiac arrest: risk stratification by anatomic substrate. Am Heart J 1993; 126:807.

Vlodaver Z, Edwards JE. Pathology of coronary atherosclerosis. Progr Cardiov Dis 1971; 14:256.

Vlodaver Z, Kahn HA, Neufeld HN. The coronary arteries in early life in three different ethnic groups. Circulation 1969; 39:541.

Vlodaver Z, Medalic I, Neufeld HN. Coronary arteries in immature monkeys. Preliminary report of the relationship to activity and diet. J Atheros Res 1968a;8:923.

Vlodaver Z, Neufeld HM. The musculo-elastic layer in the coronary arteries. A histological and hemodynamic concept. Vasc Dis 1967; 4:136.

Vlodaver Z, Neufeld HN. The coronary arteries in coarctation of the aorta. Circulation 1968b;37:449.

Vogt A, Von Essen R, Tebbe U et al. Impact of early perfusion status of the infarct-artery on short-term mortality after thrombolysis for acute myocardial infarction: retrospective analysis of four German multicenter studies. J Am Coll Cardiol 1993; 21:1391.

Voigt J, Agdal N. Lipomatous infiltration of the heart. Arch Pathol Lab Med 1982; 106:497.

Wal van der AC, Becker AE, Loos van der CM et al. Site of intimal rupture or erosion of thrombosed coronary atherosclerotic plaques is characterized by an inflammatory process irrespective of the dominant plaque morphology. Circulation 1994; 89:36.

Wal van der AC, Das PK, Berg van der DB et al. Atherosclerotic lesions in humans. In situ immunophenotypic analysis suggesting an immune mediated response. Lab Invest 1989; 61;166.

Waller BF. Pathology of new cardiovascular interventional procedures. In: Silver MD, ed. Cardiovascular Pathology. 2nd ed. New York: Churchill Livingstone Inc. 1991:1683.

Waller BF, Pinkerton CA. "Cutters, scoopers, shavers and scrapers": The importance of atherectomy devices and clinical relevance of tissue removed. J Am Coll Cardiol 1990; 15:426.

Waller BF, Roberts WC. Sudden death while running in conditioned runners aged 40 years or over. Am J Cardiol 1980; 45:1292.

Waller BF, Rothbaum DA, Pinkerton CA et al. Status of the myocardium and infarct-related coronary artery in 19 necropsy patients with acute recanalization using pharmacologic (streptokinase, r-tissue plasminogen activator), mechanical (percutaneous transluminal coronary angioplasty) or combined types of reperfusion therapy. J Am Coll Cardiol 1987; 9:785.

Wanibuchi H, Veda M, Dingermans KP et al. The response to percutaneous transluminal coronary angioplasty: an ultrastructural study of smooth muscle cells and endothelial cells. Cardiovasc Pathol 1992; 1:295.

Ware JA, Heistad DD. Platelet-endothelium interactions. N Engl J Med 1993; 328:628.

Warnes CA, Roberts WC. Sudden coronary death: comparison of patients with to those without coronary thrombus at necroscopy. Am J Cardiol 1984; 54:1206.

Warren JV. Di si dolce morte. It may be safer to be dead than alive. Circulation 1974; 50:415.

Wartman WB. Occlusion of the coronary arteries by hemorrhage into their walls. Am Heart J 1938; 15:459.

Wearn JT. The extent of the capillary bed of the heart. J Exper Med 1928; 47:273.

Webster MW, Chesebro JH, Smith HC et al. Myocardial infarction and coronary artery occlusion: a prospective 5-year angiographic study.J Am Coll Cardiol 1990; 15:218A.

Weiner HL, Swain L. Acidic fibroblast growth factor in RNA is expressed by cardiac myocytes in culture and the protein is localized to the extracellular matrix. Proc Natl Acad Sci USA 1989; 86:2683.

Weiss DL, Subswicz B, Rubenstein I. Myocardial lesions of calcium deficiency causing irreversible myocardial failure. Am J Path 1966; 48:653.

Weisse AB, Lehan PH, Ettinger PO et al. The fate of experimentally induced coronary thrombosis. Am J Cardiol 1969; 23:229.

Wenger NK, Bauer S. Coronary embolism. Review of the literature and presentation of fifteen cases. Am J Med 1958; 25:549.

White PD, Boursy AV. Translation of De Subitaneis Mortibus (on sudden deaths). New York: St. John's University Press, 1970.

Wight TN, Curwen KD, Litrenta MM et al. Effect of endothelium on glycosaminoglycan accumulation in injured rabbit aorta. Am J Path 1983; 113:156.

Wijns W, Serruys PW, Slager CJ et al. Effect of coronary occlusion during percutaneous transluminal angioplasty in humans on left ventricular chamber stiffness and regional diastolic pressure-radius relations. J Am Coll Cardiol 1986; 3:455.

Wikstrand J, Kendall M. The role of beta receptor blockade in preventing sudden death. Eur Heart J 1992; 13 (Suppl D):111.

Wikstrand J, Warnold I, Olsson G et al. Primary prevention with metopolol in patients with hypertension. Mortality results from the MAPHY study. JAMA 1988; 259:1976.

Williams DD, Amsterdam EA, Miller RR et al. Functional significance of coronary collateral vessels in patients with acute myocardial infarction: relation to pump performance, cardiogenic shock and survival. Am J Cardiol 1976; 37:345.

Willich SN, Maclure M, Mittleman M et al. Sudden cardiac death. Support for a role of triggering in causation. Circulation 1993; 87:1442.

Wilson JB. An introduction to scientific research. New York: McGraw-Hill, 1952:41.

Wilson RF, Laxson DD, Christenen RV et al. Regional differences in sympathetic reinnervation after human orthotopic cardiac transplantation. Circulation 1993; 88:165.

Wissler RW. The arterial medial cell, smooth muscle of multifunctional mesenchyme? Circulation 1967; 36:1.

Wissler RW. Current status of regression studies. In: Paoletti R, Gotto AM Jr, eds. Atherosclerosis Review. Vol 3. New York: Raven Press, 1978:213.

Wolinsky H. Effects of estrogen and progestogen treatment on the response of the aorta of male rats to hypertension. Morphological studies. Circul Res 1972; 30:341.

Wolkoff K. Ueber die Atherosklerose der Coronarterien des Herzens. Beitr Path Anat 1929; 82:555.

World Health Organization (WHO) Report: Scientific group on the pathological diagnosis of acute ischemic heart disease. Geneve:1969.

World Health Organization (WHO): Prevention of ischemic heart disease; metabolic aspect. In: Fejfar Z, Oliver MF eds. Report of a WHO symposium. 1972.

Yamagashi M, Miyatake K, Tamai J et al. Intravascular ultrasound detection of atherosclerosis at the site of focal vasospasm in angiographically normal or minimally narrowed coronary segments. J Am Coll Cardiol 1994; 23:352.

Yamamoto H, Tomoike H, Shimokawa H et al. Development of collateral function with repetitive coronary occlusion in a canine model reduces myocardial reactive hyperemia in the absence of significant coronary stenosis. Circ Res 1984; 55:623.

Yamori Y, Mano M, Nara Y et al. Cathecolamine-induced polyploidization in vascular smooth muscle cells. Circulation 1987; 75 (suppl 1)I -92.

Zamir M, Silver MD. Vasculature in the walls of human coronary arteries. Arch Pathol Lab Med 1985; 109:659.

Zerbini EJ. Coronary ligation in wounds of the heart. Report of a case in which ligation of the anterior descending branch of the left coronary artery was followed by complete recovery. J Thorac Surg 1943; 12:642.

Zhao M, Zhang H, Robinson TF et al. Profound structural alterations of the extracellular collagen matrix in postischemic dysfunctional ("stunned") but viable myocardium. J Am Coll Cardiol 1987; 10:1322.

Zimmermann ANE, Daems W, Hulsmann WC et al. Morphopathological changes of heart muscle caused by successive perfusion with calcium-free and calcium containing solutions (calcium paradox). Cardiov Res 1967; 1:201.

Zipes DP. Electrophysiological mechanism involved in ventricular fibrillation. Circulation 1975; 51-52(Suppl 3):3-120.

INDEX

Page numbers in italics denote figures (f) or tables (t).